THE NEW
MEDICAL
MARKETPLACE

THE NEW MEDICAL MARKETPLACE

A PHYSICIAN'S GUIDE

TO THE HEALTH CARE REVOLUTION

by Anne Stoline, M.D.
and Jonathan P. Weiner, Ph.D.

with Peter E. Dans, M.D., Gail Geller, M.P.H.,
and Mary G. Mussman, M.D., M.P.H.

The Johns Hopkins University Press
Baltimore and London

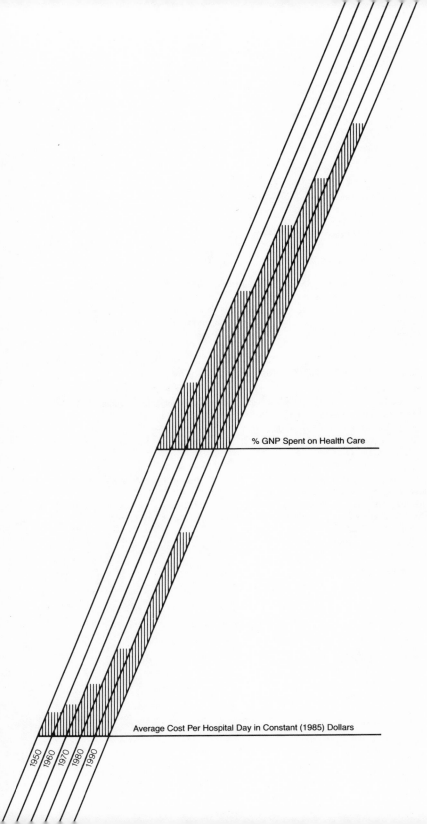

% GNP Spent on Health Care

Average Cost Per Hospital Day in Constant (1985) Dollars

1950 1960 1970 1980 1990

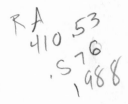

The Johns Hopkins University Press, 701 West 40th Street, Baltimore, Maryland 21211
The Johns Hopkins Press Ltd., London

The paper used in this publication meets the minimum requirements of American National
Standard for Information Sciences—Permanence of Paper for Printed Library Materials, ANSI
Z39.48-1984. ∞

LIBRARY OF CONGRESS CATALOGING-IN-PUBLICATION DATA

Stoline, Anne, 1961–
    The new medical marketplace: a physician's guide to the health care revolution / by Anne
Stoline and Jonathan Weiner, with Peter Dans, Gail Geller, and Mary Mussman.
        p.   cm.
    Bibliography: p.
    Includes index.
    ISBN 0-8018-3644-1 (alk. paper). ISBN 0-8018-3645-X (pbk. : alk. paper)
    1. Medical economics—United States.   2. Medical care, Cost of—Moral and ethical
aspects.   I. Weiner, Jonathan P.   II. Title.
    [DNLM: 1. Delivery of Health Care—economics—United States.   2. Economics, Medical—
trends—United States.   3. Health Policy—trends—United States.   W 74 S875n]
RA410.53.S76   1988
338.4'73621'0973—dc19
DNLM/DLC
for Library of Congress   87-34224
                                                                CIP

THE DEVELOPMENT OF THIS BOOK WAS SUPPORTED, IN PART, THROUGH GRANTS FROM THE NATIONAL FUND FOR MEDICAL EDUCATION AND THE W. K. KELLOGG FOUNDATION TO THE OFFICE OF MEDICAL PRACTICE EVALUATION OF THE JOHNS HOPKINS MEDICAL INSTITUTIONS

Once upon a time, the American health care system flourished in a fool's paradise of cost-plus reimbursement and bottomless budgets. No wonder consideration of cost never sullied medical education in those days! In 1975, as cost-burdened government, industry and insurers began to intrude on that paradise, the National Fund for Medical Education originated an idea: if future physicians were introduced to economic reality, the medical profession might cease to be part of the cost problem and become part of the solution. NFME challenged educators to develop innovative ways to teach medical students and residents how to give the highest quality of care at the least cost within ethical constraints. "Care, Cost, and Conscience" paraphrases that challenge. The Fund is proud to have contributed to the creation of this book. *The New Medical Marketplace* is an invaluable guide for the practitioners who must blaze new trails into an uncertain future.

John Gordon Freymann, M.D.
President Emeritus
National Fund for Medical Education

CONTENTS

FOREWORD

The scientific and technical aspects of medical practice have been undergoing a continuous revolution for more than half a century, but until recently the system for delivering medical care in the United States and the position of the physician within that system had not changed very much. Students and new physicians could concentrate on acquiring the medical information and skills they needed, secure in the knowledge that they would be entering a stable medical care system in which they would be free to practice their profession as they saw fit, under whichever arrangements they chose. The role of the physician as the center of power in the system was accepted without question.

All that has now changed. An economic crisis has developed which is reshaping the structure of American health care, profoundly affecting the way doctors work. With the problem of cost have also come new problems, of access to care and the maintenance of quality. Social, political, and legal forces impinge on the practice of medicine as never before, and physicians confront ethical and economic problems undreamed of even a decade ago. These, in turn, have necessitated changes in style of practice. Solo, fee-for-service practice dominated the scene until recently, but new arrangements are now coming to the fore, and very soon most young physicians will be practicing in some kind of group setting, often on a salaried basis. In many cases, physicians are being asked to share financial risks with insurers or are being hired directly by insurers to provide care to beneficiaries, thus creating new and disturbing conflicts of interest between doctors and patients. Even in fee-for-service practice, competitive economic pressures have encouraged entrepreneurial behavior among many physicians, creating a commercial climate in medicine that has rarely if ever been seen before.

This revolution seems to have taken most of the medical profession by surprise. Immersed in their own practices, relatively uninformed about the gathering social and economic forces, physicians did not see the handwriting on the wall, were not prepared for what happened, and could do little more than watch in frustration as their influence waned and the control of their future was gradually taken over by others. Not surprisingly, their level of unhappiness is high and their expressions of dissatisfaction with the present state of medical practice abound.

But physicians need not be pawns or simply react to changes initiated by others. I believe there is still time for them to take constructive actions that would defend traditional professional values and promote the interests of their patients. To do this, however, they will need to learn the objective facts about, and understand the social and economic forces behind, the current health care revolution. That is why this book is so important. In clear and succinct style, Stoline and Weiner, and their colleagues, take the reader on a rapid tour of the changing medical scene. They show why change was inevitable, and they explain the inadequacies and contradictions of our present nonsystem. Reading this book one cannot fail to see the problems and gain insight into their possible solutions. No detailed answers are provided, but most of the ingredients for intelligent policy-making are here.

This book ought to be part of a required course for medical students, who now are given lamentably little education about the new social climate in which they will be practicing. It could also be read with much benefit by physicians in training or in established practices who want to understand what has been happening to them, and why.

Of course, this understanding ought to be followed by thoughtful and constructive action. That will require more collective initiative and moral conviction than we have seen so far, but no useful action is possible without the kind of insights provided here. I am enthusiastic about *The New Medical Marketplace* because it provides information which is needed by physicians at this time but which is almost impossible to find so neatly and attractively packaged in one place. If enough doctors and medical students read this book and ponder its lessons, we might see the medical profession begin serious efforts to improve the present state of affairs. Such efforts, if based on the clear vision afforded by books like this one, might even have a chance of succeeding.

Arnold S. Relman, M.D.
Editor, *New England Journal of Medicine*

THE NEW
MEDICAL
MARKETPLACE

CHAPTER 1

THE NEW WAY OF MEDICINE

Huge changes have taken place in recent years in the way health care in the United States is organized and provided, in the way medical and hospital services are paid for, and in the influence of government and business in the marketplace for health services. Medical practitioners often react to these changes with bewilderment, resentment, and above all anxiety. Practicing physicians worry that the changes will compromise the quality of health care and alter their professional relationship with patients. Medical students and residents worry about where the profession is heading. This book, addressed chiefly to readers in the medical professions, explains what has happened and why, and offers guidance for coping with the many challenges the new system offers to medical practice, financing, and ethics.

The revolution in health care was set in motion over a decade ago by a rapid inflation of expenditures.

By 1990, U.S. medical care expenditures are expected to reach $2,500 per capita—a total expenditure of $650 billion accounting for more than 11 percent of the nation's annual gross national product.

No nation has ever spent anywhere near this much on health care, and many contend that no nation ever can without short-changing other critical sectors of society. The escalation of costs has prompted an evaluation of the benefits obtained from our massive commitment of resources to health care.

In 1985, U.S. per-capita health care costs were two and one-half times those of Great Britain, yet average life expectancy and most other health indicators were comparable across the two countries.

For these reasons, today's physician practices in an environment with an unprecedented emphasis on the fiscal bottom line. Among other things, physicians must justify most major clinical decisions to third-party payers and managers. The one-to-one interaction between a patient and a "private" practitioner where the fees are paid directly by the patient or a distant insurance company is now nearly nonexistent; the rules of the game have changed. Today, the health care system is characterized by a complex latticework of financial relationships in which complete, unnegotiated fee-for-service payment is the exception, not the rule. The new triumvirate of American health care financing—government, employers, and insurance companies—who pay over 75 percent of the bill are increasingly using their buying power to restrain the upward spiral in costs.

As recently as ten years ago, an understanding of health care financing and organization was considered unnecessary for most physicians. Today, in the new medical marketplace, this is no longer true; in addition to clinical knowledge and ethical concerns, cost has become a major variable in the provider-patient equation. Physicians trained to put a patient's medical welfare above all else now find themselves obligated to balance clinical considerations not only against that patient's financial welfare but against society's apparent judgment that health care expenditures in general are too high. Small wonder that so many clinicians feel caught between the new rules of the game and their responsibility to uphold the professional code of ethics.

Under the financial incentives of the traditional fee-for-service practice, when doctors and hospitals for the most part were paid whatever they requested, many believed that patients were at risk of too much care. Some surgical procedures such as hysterectomies, prostatectomies, and tonsillectomies vary in frequency up to six-fold across populations or regions. Critics have suggested that this variation is due as much to the financial needs of hospitals and surgeons as to the clinical needs of patients.

As a further indication of variability, Medicare data since 1965 show that hospital length-of-stay for the same condition consistently has been 2.5 days longer in the northeastern states than in the west.

This wide variation of "accepted" practice undermines the position of physicians who would wish to be left alone to set their own standards. Yet while regulating the performance of practitioners may be appropriate from a cost-cutting perspective, from the perspective of patient care the loss of the physician's autonomy in clinical decision making could be catastrophic. Medicare's new system of prospective payment—with hospitals receiving a fixed payment per admission—now places patients at risk of receiving less care than needed, rather than more. The logic of this and other mechanisms of cost containment—to trim away unnecessary care—is simple; what is not so simple is the identification of which services are excessive and which are necessary. The process of making clinical decisions is, and always will be, replete with uncertainty, and the ultimate responsibility for the results of these decisions, many of which can affect patients profoundly, rests with the physician—not the payer or policymaker.

Balancing cost containment with the best interests of the patient always will be difficult, but the process could be made more rational. As the growth of medical technology offers new tests and treatments, physicians, faced with what has been called the "technological imperative," have too commonly incorporated them into practice in an additive rather than integrative way. Test ordering as a rote behavior has contributed to the escalation of health care expenditures. So, too, has the increase of malpractice litigation, inducing some physicians to alter their clinical decisions in a style of "defensive" medicine. In today's era of cost control, such practices have contributed to what seems an underlying distrust of physicians and other providers by third-party payers. Gone is the presumption that what the physician chooses to do is correct unless proven wrong. The current system is pushing medical practitioners inexorably in the direction of making conscious tradeoffs between cost and care.

As a result of social and economic pressures, the real income of physicians began to decline in 1983. The principal causes of this cut in earnings are a decrease in rates of reimbursement, competition from an increasing supply of young physicians, and a shift of physicians into salaried positions.

Recent surveys indicate that over half of American physicians now receive some or all of their income in the form of a basic salary.

Many physicians are entangled in a complex web of contracts with health maintenance organizations (HMOs), preferred provider organizations (PPOs), hospital joint ventures, and insurers who "manage" the care or services they provide. Traditional education has left them woefully unprepared for the negotiations such contracts require.

In California and some other states, over half of all practicing physicians now contract with one or more HMOs or PPOs.

This involvement with organized "corporate" providers of care raises many issues. Health care administrators increasingly view clinicians as simply another organizational resource rather than, as in past eras, independent professionals around which the organization revolves. Equally significant, under HMO arrangements physicians usually benefit when the organization's capitation-based revenue is higher than expenditures. Moreover, the physician is often an investor in care facilities; investors always profit when revenues exceed costs. Financial incentives and pressures are shifting—largely toward the provision of less care.

Although the new medical marketplace has been imposed on the profession primarily from without, physicians are not exactly "innocent bystanders." The cost containment problem was caused, to a significant degree, by their own practices and conventions. Yet it is not too late for physicians and other providers to influence the ongoing health care revolution. Indeed, it is essential that their voices be heard on a wide range of critical issues. The same is true of health care consumers, whether individual patients or community-level officials and organizations.

The material in this primer has been presented as simply as possible without misrepresenting the complex issues at stake. Moreover, a variety of perspectives have been incorporated. The authors and contributors include a recent medical school graduate, a health policy and management specialist with particular experience in the design and evaluation of health care delivery systems, a seasoned internist involved in studies of clinical decisions and technologies, a medical practice analyst with interests in medical ethics and medical education, and a pediatrician who at the onset of this project was in her residency. The authors also had the considerable benefit of advice from a range of consultants within the Johns Hopkins Medical Institutions, people expert in the areas of decision analysis, medical ethics, health economics, nursing, and medical history. Although the text that follows is written by medical people for "the profession" of physicians, medical students, and other clinical workers and trainees, it is addressed also to others with deep interests in America's emergent health care delivery system. Policymakers, health care administrators, corporate benefit managers, insurance executives, and last, but certainly not least, activated consumers of medical services can find clarification of the many complex issues treated in this book. May it ease the new way for all.

CHAPTER 2

HISTORICAL BACKGROUND

s Alvin Tarlov writes: "The medical objectives of an era emanate from two formative influences. The first relates to the state of the art in the medical science of the period, which provides an understanding of disease processes and therapeutic modalities for successful intervention. The second is society's expectation of health care. These two influences coalesce to make explicit the social purpose of the system. Each era of medical objectives builds on the last. The eras overlap considerably" (1983, p. 1239).

Most societal change is evolutionary and incremental. An overall view of society's functions and purposes—in Kuhn's term, a paradigm—is widely accepted. As its implications are increasingly explored, progress of sorts occurs, but with it comes a kind of dissonance or instability owing to inevitable shifts in societal beliefs and patterns of living. This instability leads to more or less modest changes in the paradigm: new ways are gradually accepted as former beliefs are modified or replaced. In contrast, the development of an entirely new paradigm, for society or a facet of it, may lead to revolutionary change. There is a "watershed" period during which a new paradigm gains acceptance, and this is followed by an era of relative stability until another paradigm appears.

The U.S. health care system is currently undergoing a revolutionary transition. Because its causes originated in past events, the present revolution can be better understood when the circumstances leading to its occurrence are considered.

Entering the Twentieth Century

The Industrial Revolution of the 1830s brought much of the United States population into the cities in search of steady employment and a better life, only to have their dreams shattered by the harsh reality of poor housing, inadequate food, unclean water, and unsafe working conditions. Life on the farm, though somewhat better, was far from idyllic; not only farmers but their wives and children did backbreaking work for long hours for very little return. For most Americans, poor sewage disposal and crowded living conditions facilitated the spread of infectious diseases, which were the major cause of sickness and death in the nineteenth century. The average life expectancy in 1900 was only 47 years, owing in large part to high infant and child mortality.

Before the turn of the century, the predominant government involvement in health care was in the military. In 1775 funds were authorized to build a hospital for the Revolutionary Army. In 1798 the Marine Hospital Service (forerunner of the U.S. Public Health Service) was created to care for merchant seamen who contracted communicable—mainly sexually transmitted—diseases during their travels. Although federal government involvement in health care for civilians began to expand at this time, most medical care spending went toward city, county, and state public health programs. Health policy focused on environmental and community health.

The American Public Health Association, founded in 1872, worked to establish community health standards, and civic reformers clamored for changes. Some changes, like improvements in housing and food, were only indirectly disease-related, but were very directly related to citizens' health. A number of legislative reforms were passed, including the first Food and Drug Act; municipal health departments were created and visiting nurse services were provided. Most important were programs to provide clean water supplies and proper waste disposal. These actions were instrumental in improving social conditions and average life expectancy. In the words of Oliver Wendell Holmes, a prominent physician of the late nineteenth century, "The bills of mortality are more affected by drainage than this or that medical practice" (Ackernecht 1982, p. 210).

Medical practice remained unsophisticated at the turn of the century, primarily because disease models as we know them today had little currency. Much important scientific research had been done and hints of a revolution to come were evident, but there was no medical profession as such to respond to the new research. For example, though microbiology was gaining acceptance as a discipline thanks to pioneer researchers like Pasteur and Semmelweis, the notion of antisepsis was slow to take hold; even at the turn of the century, most surgeons still operated with bare hands.

There were only a few effective compounds in the pharmacopoeia of the 1890s, notably digitalis, morphine, and the smallpox vaccine. In an address to the Massachusetts Medical Society, Holmes exempted opium, wine, and anesthetics, and then stated: "I firmly believe that if the whole materia medica, *as now used*, could be sunk to the bottom of the sea, it would be all the better for mankind—and all the worse for the fishes" (Evans 1978, p. 439).

Schools with differing approaches to medical care—among them allopathy, osteopathy, homeopathy, botany, and eclecticism—coexisted in a state of fierce rivalry. Prospective students faced a bewildering choice among some 160 medical schools; few of these schools required a high school diploma for admission or provided students with any grounding in science, and many were in business chiefly for profit. The typical medical school program lasted two years and consisted mainly of lectures. Patient contact was a neglected aspect of most programs. The American Medical Association (AMA), established in 1847, was composed primarily of allopathic practitioners.*

Most physicians used what medical knowledge they had to benefit the sick, but some practitioners were less scrupulous.

---

*The term allopathy, or "other" therapy, drew its label mainly in contrast to homeopathy, or "like" therapy. In homeopathy the belief was that "like cured like"; small amounts of drugs that in larger amounts actually cause a disease were used to fight it. That approach relied on eliciting the body's own defensive responses. The allopathic philosophy (the predominant form of medicine to this day) was based on creating a second condition incompatible with the patient's presenting disease.

Since no laws prohibited false claims on drug labels, bottled preparations labeled as a cure for cancer could legally be sold and were; and since narcotics had not yet been brought under government control, "soothing syrups" for babies contained morphine, many preparations contained cocaine, and the active ingredient in a popular concoction known as Lydia Pinkham's Tonic was ethanol.

As might be expected, some self-styled healers, less politely known as quacks, used consumer ignorance to profit financially. "*Quacks* is short for *quacksalvers*, or people who applied salves of quicksilver (mercury). 'Quacking out' [or advertising] in the marketplace, they stood in contrast to regular physicians who weren't supposed to advertise themselves. The essence of quackery was retailing 'secret remedies,' often called 'patent medicines,' which meant not that the formula itself was patented but that the name was trademarked" (Shorter 1985, pp. 69–70).

Regular physicians also often misrepresented their wares, though from better motives. Having little but compassion to offer a sick patient, but aware that charisma could sometimes transform a worthless nostrum into effective treatment, they regularly wrote detailed prescriptions for inactive compounds and urged them on their patients. "The contents were a deep mystery, and intended to be a mystery. . . . The purpose of this kind of therapy was essentially reassurance. . . . They were placebos, and they had been the principal mainstay of medicine, the sole technology, for so long a time—millennia—that they had the incantatory power of religious ritual" (Thomas 1983, p. 15).

The type of health care patients received was determined by their ability to pay and their geographic location. In the cities wealthy patients were treated in their homes by private physicians. Poor people in the cities, if able and willing to leave their sickbeds, commonly obtained free services from outdoor dispensaries funded by the city and private charities. Those who stayed at home either received visits from a dispensary physician or relied on folk healing methods. Beginning at the turn of the century, publicly funded visiting nurses became an important source of professional home care for the poor, especially for children and pregnant women.

THE PEOPLE'S

COMMON SENSE

MEDICAL ADVISER

IN PLAIN ENGLISH;

OR,

MEDICINE SIMPLIFIED.

BY

R. V. PIERCE, M. D.

ONE OF THE STAFF OF CONSULTING PHYSICIANS AND SURGEONS
AT THE INVALIDS' HOTEL AND SURGICAL INSTITUTE, AND
PRESIDENT OF THE WORLD'S DISPENSARY
MEDICAL ASSOCIATION.

SIXTY-FOURTH EDITION.

Two Million and Fifty Thousand.

*Carefully Revised by the Author, assisted by his full Staff of Asso-
ciate Specialists in Medicine and Surgery, the Faculty of
the Invalids' Hotel and Surgical Institute.*

PRINTED AND PUBLISHED AT THE WORLD'S DISPENSARY PRINTING
OFFICE AND BINDERY,

BUFFALO, N. Y., U. S. A.

INTRODUCTORY WORDS.

The profession of medicine is no *sinecure;* its labors are constant, its toils unremitting, its cares unceasing. The physician is expected to meet the grim monster, "break the jaws of death, and pluck the spoil out of his teeth." *His* ear is ever attentive to entreaty, and within his faithful breast are concealed the disclosures of the suffering. Success may elate him, as conquest flushes the victor. Honors are lavished upon the brave soldiers who, in the struggle with the foe, have covered themselves with glory, and returned victorious from the field of battle; but how much more brilliant is the achievement of those who overwhelm disease, that common enemy of mankind, whose victims are numbered by millions! Is it meritorious in the physician to modestly veil his discoveries, regardless of their importance? If he have light, why hide it from the world? Truth should be made as universal and health-giving as sunlight. We say, give light to all who are in darkness, and a remedy to the afflicted everywhere.

REMEDIES FOR DISEASE.

Dr. Pierce's Golden Medical Discovery. In addition to the alterative properties combined in this compound, it possesses important tonic qualities. While the Favorite Prescription exerts a tonic influence upon the digestive and nutritive functions, the Golden Medical Discovery acts upon the excretory glands. Besides, it tends to retard unusual waste and expenditure. This latter remedy tones, sustains, and, at the same time regulates the functions. While increasing the discharge of noxious elements accumulated in the system, it promptly arrests the wastes arising from debility, and the unusual breaking down of the cells incident to quick decline. It stimulates the liver to secrete, changes the sallow complexion, and transforms the listless invalid into a vigorous and healthy being. At the same time, it checks the rapid disorganization of the tissues and their putrescent change, while it sustains the vital processes. It is, therefore, an indispensable remedy in the treatment of many diseases.

Dr. Pierce's Pleasant Pellets, being entirely vegetable in their composition, operate without disturbance to the system, diet, or occupation. Put up in glass vials. Always fresh and reliable. As *a laxative, alterative,* or gently acting but searching *cathartic,* these little Pellets give the most perfect satisfaction. Sick Headache, Bilious Headache, Dizziness, Constipation, Indigestion, Bilious Attacks, and all derangements of the stomach and bowels, are promptly relieved and permanently cured by the use of Dr. Pierce's Pleasant Pellets. In explanation of the remedial power of these Pellets over so great a variety of diseases, it may truthfully be said that their action upon the system is universal, not a gland or tissue escaping their sanative influence.

Dr. Pierce's Favorite Prescription. The Favorite Prescription, in addition to those properties already described, likewise combines tonic properties. In consequence of the never ceasing activities of the bodily organs, the system requires support, something to permanently exalt its actions. In all cases of debility, the Favorite Prescription tranquilizes the nerves, tones up the organs and increases their vigor, and strengthens the system. Directions for use accompany every bottle.

Excerpts from Dr. Pierce's widely read consumer guide, printed in 1895. His Institute specialized in mail-order dispensing.

In 1873 there were fewer than 200 hospitals in the United States. Most were in large cities, and approximately one-third provided care for the mentally ill. The word "hospital" derives from the Latin words *hospes*, for "host," and *hospitalis*, meaning "of a guest." The typical hospital of this era *was* little more than a guest house for people who lacked family or the financial resources to sustain them through an illness. Hospitals were also commonly used for the isolation of patients with communicable infectious diseases. A patient with enough money could be admitted to a pay ward or private room, but most were cared for in large charity wards. All in all, the hospital at the turn of the century held little advantage over home care. With its limited techniques, surgery could be performed as easily at home as in the hospital, and the risk of being infected by another patient was avoided at home. Also, of course, patients preferred to be at home during convalescence.

Many hospitals were run by religious orders, which held expenses to a minimum. Operating a hospital was viewed as charity work, and expenses were often subsidized by affluent citizens. Physicians and nurses donated their skills to such hospitals, arranging to visit the wards several times a week. Because of their mission to the poor and the poverty of their patient population, few charged for their services.

Physicians at the turn of the century usually had offices in their own homes. Many traveled on horseback or by buggy to make house calls, carrying all equipment available to them in a single bag. Despite the abundance of medical schools, physicians were in short supply in many regions, and workloads were particularly heavy in rural areas.

In 1870 a house call cost 50–75 cents, an office call 25 cents. The average hospital stay cost only about a dollar per day. Insurance to pay for medical expenses had been instituted in Europe during the Industrial Revolution, but was not yet common in the United States, except for some immigrant union workers in large cities. Financial transactions between the patient and his physician or the hospital were typically direct, with some bills being paid in produce, livestock, or services, particularly in rural areas. Most turn-of-the-century physicians were not affluent.

Many physicians settled permanently in one location and cared for patients—often more than one generation of a family—from birth to death. The personal relationships that developed gave such physicians a respected place in the community, and they were consulted on a wide variety of issues. *Indeed, a romanticized image of the seemingly selfless and inexhaustible practitioner, dating from this era, has remained as our standard for professional dedication.* Physicians benefit from this image to this day in the respect they are accorded. Yet the very attachment to such an idealized image has made it difficult for physicians and others to be objective about changes in the delivery of medical care. Changes occur anyway, of course, but not all are quickly accepted.

From 1900 to World War II

In parallel with the rising importance of the machine model in the industrial world, medicine moved out of the prescientific era during the early 1900s. Physicians began to view the body as a composite of individual systems, systems that "could be examined and treated without the rest of the body being affected" (Berliner 1975, p. 576). This shift in thinking paved the way for the advent of medical specialization and for research focusing on pathophysiologic processes; there was a decreased emphasis on the social causes of disease.

Beginning at the turn of the century, rapid advances were made in diagnosis and therapy. X-rays had been recently discovered and were soon used for diagnosis. The electrocardiogram was developed in the early 1900s. New pharmaceuticals were discovered and entered general use. In 1910 arsphenamine was introduced for the treatment of syphilis, and in the 1920s the discovery of insulin made the treatment of diabetes possible. The development of the sulfa drugs (1935) and penicillin (1941) provided the first effective treatments against many infectious diseases. Effective therapy for asthma and initial breakthroughs toward understanding the allergic process also date from this era.

For surgical patients, effective anesthetics became readily available and the widespread acceptance of antiseptic techniques minimized bacterial growth. The discovery of the four major blood

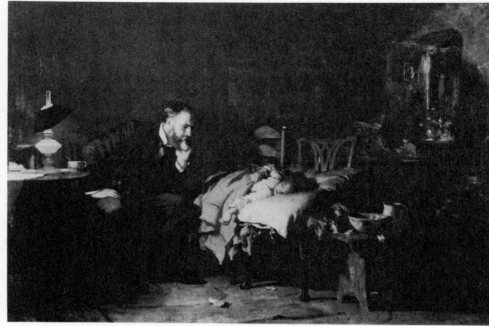

Sir Luke Fildes (1844–1927), *The Doctor*. Oil on canvas, 1891. (Source: The Tate Gallery, London.)

groups in 1901 permitted safer blood transfusions. These improvements in turn led to great advances in surgical technique. In the early 1900s several operations that were experimental and highly dangerous only a few years earlier became commonplace. Surgical mortality rates initially rose, but as pioneering surgeons became more proficient at the new techniques the rates soon declined.

For example, prior to 1890 appendicitis was treated by allowing the inflamed appendix to rupture, form an abscess, and wall itself off before the abdomen was opened. The first successful appendectomy was performed in 1890. Over time, as knowledge of the technique spread and surgeons became skilled at performing it, appendectomy became the new standard of practice. Over a seventeen-year time span, from 1893 to 1910, mortality from appendectomies dropped from 26 percent to 2 percent.

Knowledge increased tremendously, which allowed "diseases to be treated as universal entities rather than as individual afflictions different for everyone" (Berliner 1975, p. 576). The explosion of therapeutic advances increased the volume of medical care and heightened its complexity. Allopathic physicians thoroughly incorporated scientific attitudes into their medical care, and from this point forth declared themselves to be the only legitimate medical practitioners.

As a result of these changes, the personalized, holistic approach to patient care began to decline during this era; the patient was removed from the social context of his affliction, and was "thought of almost as an abstraction" (ibid.). Whereas patients and physicians had formerly viewed disease similarly, the physician's scientific knowledge now created a disparity between their views. Thus, for example, whereas people might continue to believe that they could "catch a cold" when their feet got wet, more and more physicians knew that colds were caused by viruses and bacteria.

But all this took time, and even decades later practitioners were still without cures for many common conditions, as we learn from Lewis Thomas, who accompanied his physician father on house calls in the 1920s. "The general drift of his conversation was intended to make clear to me, early on, the aspect of medicine that troubled him most all through his professional life; there were so many people needing help, and so little that he could do for any of them. It was necessary for him to be available, and to make all these calls at their homes, but I was not to have the idea that he could do anything much to change the course of their illnesses" (1983, p. 13).

While established practitioners were only beginning to feel its effects, scientific progress was having a significant impact on medical education. The modern physician needed a greater range of skills than the old-fashioned medical education could supply. The Association of American Medical Colleges, founded in 1876, had begun to develop stricter standards for medical school members, but far more sweeping changes were needed. They came

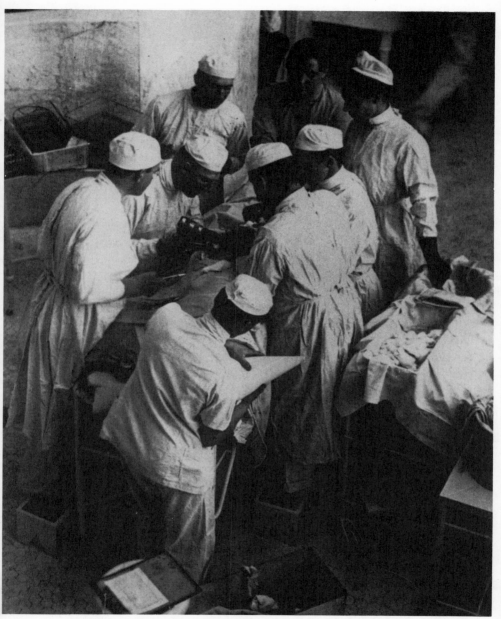

Surgical operation at the Johns Hopkins Hospital, Baltimore, 1904. (Source: The Chesney Medical Archives of the Johns Hopkins Medical Institutions.) Dr. William S. Halstead is the lead surgeon in the center.

with the publication in 1910 of the Flexner Report (so called after its main author, Abraham Flexner), which codified a general shift in society's approach to educating physicians. Based on a study sponsored by the Rockefeller and Carnegie Foundations, the Flexner Report has been called the single most important document in the history of American health care.

Two years (preferably four) of undergraduate college education, including courses in the basic sciences, became the requirement for admission to medical school. This requirement made it much harder for a relatively poor person to obtain a medical education and thus altered the social structure of the profession. In addition, from that point on all medical schools took a common approach to the study of the patient and disease: the AMA and allopathic medicine had emerged the victors of the competition among sects.

The association of medical schools with universities also dates from this time. Medical schools developed into research centers specializing in the application of sophisticated technology, and the role of patient care was reduced in importance. The duration of the medical school program increased to four years. The number of medical schools had already been decreasing, and as schools that could not meet the new standards closed, the decline in both the number of schools and the number of their graduates continued (see Figure 1).

For a number of years there was no serious shortage of physicians, and the old system remained essentially in effect. Shorter describes the typical physician of the pre-antibiotic era as possessing "almost courtly good manners," and adds that "Around 1930, 56 percent of all GPs made [house calls]. They were frequent during an episode of illness and accumulated to an impression of caring" (1985, p. 209). Eventually, however, the transformation of medical education caused a reduction in the supply of practitioners. As Figure 1 shows, the number of medical schools and the physician-to-population ratio both reached a plateau during this time period.

Although the concept of physicians practicing jointly in a group was introduced by the Mayo family in Minnesota in the late nineteenth century, most physicians in the 1920s and 1930s

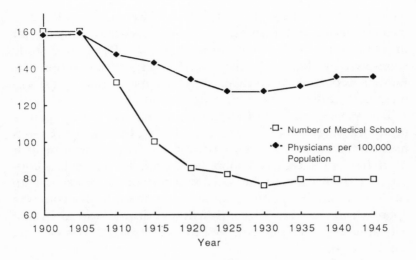

Fig. 1. Medical schools and physician manpower, 1900–1945. (Source: Fein 1962.)

practiced solo; less than one in a hundred practiced in a group of three or more. But the frequency of house calls began to decline. Not only did the lower physician-to-population ratio make them impractical for overworked practitioners, but increasingly the apparatus of adequate medical care was too complex to be transported in a bag.

Scientific advances had only begun to affect the patient-practitioner encounter outside the hospital. Within the hospital, however, much changed during this period as doctors began to require new equipment, services, and support personnel. Introducing the latest technology benefited both the hospital and the physician: the former because it attracted physicians and patients, the latter because it enabled him to practice up-to-date medicine. Diagnostic laboratories and radiology services were added in the early decades of the twentieth century, and aseptic surgical suites also became common during this time.

As it became apparent that good outcomes could result from hospital treatment, people became more willing to stay in the hospital. As a government commission reported, "The removal of the death-house stigma from the hospital was probably the most important factor in influencing the change in the public attitude toward the institution" (Commission on Hospital Care 1947, p. 49).

Soon the hospital eclipsed the home, for both wealthy and poor patients, as the preferred site for treating serious illness. The presence of illness replaced poverty as the basis for hospital admission, and the daily inpatient census came to represent a greater cross-section of the community. When this happened, the hospital became a community asset, and as such a focus of local support and pride. By the 1920s more than two-thirds of patients were paying at least some portion of the bill for care they received. As more affluent people used the hospital and were able to pay for their medical care, hospitals began to operate from a patient revenue base instead of relying chiefly on philanthropy. Still, most physicians only charged those who could pay and donated their services to those who could not.

Partly as a result of hospitals' increasing complexity, hospital charges rose; the costs of new advances were included in medical care bills. Average length of stay decreased dramatically: in part because hospitals were no longer used exclusively for long-term housing for indigent patients, but more importantly because scientific advances led to early cures of some diseases that had hitherto been left to run their natural course. Because length of stay decreased and costs increased, average costs per day increased over 200 percent from 1900 to 1930, and another 38 percent between 1930 and 1940 (Table 1).

Table 1 **Hospital Costs and Length of Stay, 1900–1944**

Year	Average costs per admission	Average length of stay (days)	Average costs per day
1900	$38	32	$1.19
1930	48	13	3.70
1940	56	11	5.09
1944	65	10	6.50

Source: Commission on Hospital Care 1947, p. 545.

When it became possible for hospitals to be run profitably, entrepreneurs were encouraged to build them, and the number of hospital beds increased substantially during this time. Population growth and the increased effectiveness of hospital care also contributed to this trend. Although the Great Depression led to a decrease in the 1930s, by 1941 there were over four times as many hospital beds as in 1909.

Socioeconomic conditions also influenced the course of development of the health care industry during this era. During the Depression years, hospitals and physicians were unable to collect fees from unemployed patients. Many people forewent elective procedures, and many chose to stay at home during an illness instead of seeking hospital care. Large numbers requested charity care, and hospital debts consequently increased. After decades of unprecedented growth, the limited flow of dollars put considerable strain on health care providers and the delivery system.

Public hospitals obtained enough government funding to remain open despite their bad debts, but proprietary hospitals, many of them founded during the booming economy of the 1920s, were hard hit. In an effort to remain financially viable in the face of decreased occupancy rates, such hospitals decreased charges, reduced employee wages, appealed to philanthropic sources of funding, and closed beds; and some limited admissions to emergency cases only. Even so, many proprietary hospitals did not survive, and the relative glut of hospital beds was reduced.

With rising medical care costs and an unstable economy, people turned to health insurance as a way of minimizing the risk of financial hardship in case of serious illness. The health insurance industry, a multi-billion-dollar giant today, grew from humble beginnings in 1929. In that year the first group health insurance plan was started in Baylor, Texas, where some 1,500 schoolteachers were enrolled in a plan that formed the basis for the Blue Cross Insurance Company. For $6 per year, enrollees received the benefit of 21 days of hospitalization coverage.

By assuring payment for a hospital stay, health insurance benefited both hospitals and patients. Thus, although ostensibly created primarily to assist the patient, health insurance was also a direct outcome of the financial crisis experienced by the hospital sector during the Depression. Some years later, insurance programs were developed (eventually called Blue Shield) to cover physicians' professional services.

Another important development was the establishment of the Veterans Administration, which offered World War I veterans treatment of service-related injuries or diseases at government expense. *This was an important turning point in the history of health policy: the first time (outside of a war situation) that total medical care for a designated group of entitled persons became a public-sector responsibility.* A precedent was set for broader measures in the future.

The composition of society changed in other ways during this era. The early 1900s brought a wave of immigrants to the United States, most of whom found employment in unskilled, poorly paid jobs. Also many Americans of all origins lost their employment during the Depression. Whereas more affluent citizens could purchase health insurance and often did so, the poor could not; and what with the physician shortage and expensive hospital bills, their needs for health care were inadequately met. Figure 2 graphs family income against physician contacts in the early years of the Depression. Note that the wealthiest Americans received more than twice as much care as the poorest.

As charity care moved from the realm of moral responsibility to become a social concern, the federal government sought to bring poor citizens under a new umbrella of limited protection. The first major effort of this type in the health field was the Sheppard-Towner Act of 1921, which provided grants to the states for maternal and child health programs. Although its objectives were not significantly different from those of the popular child labor legislation of the time, the bill was controversial, particularly among the medical community: "Many physicians opposed it. They claimed that there would be undue interference in state affairs and regimentation of medical practice" (Anderson 1985, p. 93).

During the 1930s access to care again became an issue. In 1927 the Committee on the Costs of Medical Care was formed to look into what many felt to be excessive health care costs and to ex-

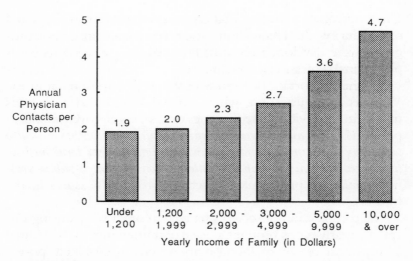

Fig. 2. Access to physicians is influenced by patient income, 1928–1931. (Source: Committee on the Costs of Medical Care 1932.)

plore ways of subsidizing health care for the poor. The comprehensiveness and foresight of this committee's recommendations had considerable impact on national health policy. The Social Security Act of 1935 incorporated some of them; others were not adopted until decades later.

Another government group, the Committee on Economic Security, was appointed in 1934 to "recommend legislation for a program 'against misfortunes which cannot be wholly eliminated in this man-made world of ours.' One of the issues to be considered by the committee was the problem of personal health services" (ibid., pp. 109–110).

Still a third government group, the Technical Committee on Medical Care, further broadened the scope of health policy by recommending grants to states for mandatory health insurance, expanded public health programs, medical care for welfare recipients, children's health care, federal permanent disability insurance, and grants for hospital construction. These recommendations were made in a proposal sent to Congress in 1939. No action was taken during World War II, but within the next twenty years all the committee's recommendations except mandatory health insurance were enacted into law.

Expenditures on health care were systematically tallied starting in 1946, and were estimated retrospectively as far back as 1929. In 1929 the country spent an estimated $3.5 billion on health care, or 3.5 percent of the gross national product. During the Depression years spending for health care decreased, reaching a low point of less than $2 billion in 1933. It increased from that year on, and by 1935 totaled some $2.9 billion or 4.0 percent of the by then somewhat shrunken gross national product.

During the New Deal years of the 1930s and 1940s, many politicians and social reformers felt that if the private sector could not provide health insurance to the masses, the government should. Extensive debates were held on the merits of national health insurance. Since any such legislation would have cut insurance companies out of the health insurance business, the growing insurance industry exerted itself to increase enrollment in private-sector health plans.

The medical profession also resisted increased government involvement in health care. What was to grow into a long history of AMA-government conflict began with the AMA's official opposition to the Sheppard-Towner Act. While acknowledging the financial advantages of private insurance and public subsidies to both patients and providers, physicians desired to maintain control over the medical care process. In particular, they did not want third-party payers to set reimbursement rates: they wanted to set these rates themselves. They were moved to some extent by sheer self-interest, but to some extent also by an unwillingness to give up the myth of the benevolent and wise solo practitioner:

Most doctors who opposed the cooperative reforms genuinely believed in the traditional ideals of individualism and freedom for the doctor and patient. Despite the scientific, professional, and economic changes which had swept over the medical profession since 1900, these men were committed to the idealized and emotionalized image of the rural general practitioner as the true representative of medical practice. Just as many industrialists of these years tended to deny real conditions and look upon themselves as benevolent partners with their employees in society's productive processes, many doctors identified themselves with the self-sacrificing and largely mythical GP of earlier decades. Somehow he, despite the fact that he carried almost all his tools in his little black bag and kept his accounts in his head, supplied the best type of medical care to his patients. And it was he who, by fulfilling his role of family doctor, by preserving the doctor-patient relationship, and by caring for the poor and unfortunate without payment or complaint, upheld the finest traditions of professional service. (Hirshfield 1970, pp. 34–35)

In this era the house call remained the emblem of professional dedication even as new technologies such as antibiotics and vaccines were demonstrating their superior effectiveness. But the practitioner's influence on the larger aspects of health care was on the wane. The new era could no longer be denied: despite physicians' efforts to maintain control of the health care industry, the influence of private insurers and politicians had begun to increase.

From World War II Through 1978

During World War II the Office of Scientific Research and Development was a unit of the military infrastructure. Among the projects coordinated by this office was the development of the atom bomb. After the war, the federal government transferred financial support from this agency to the domain of medical research.

The National Institutes of Health (NIH) has existed, in several different forms, since 1887. In 1944 Congress gave the NIH "general legislative authority to conduct research" (Spingarn 1976, p. 22). Strong financial backing of the NIH began after the war and continued through the 1960s: "The medical research renaissance . . . flowered in Bethesda [Maryland] during the 1950s and 1960s. Fact and legend mingle here, but it is true that a combination of circumstances then made NIH the great and productive leader among the world's health research institutions. An expanding economy, a favorable political ambience, a consensus stemming largely from World War II technological success that scientific research can pay off big, and a set of remarkably effective health leaders in both public and private sectors, all worked smoothly in the Institutes' behalf" (ibid., p. 5).

In part as a result of such public and private support, medical science continued to advance in this era. Research efforts in oncology focused on surgery, radiation, and chemotherapy. Vaccines were developed to counter polio and tuberculosis. Pharmacological treatment of mental illness began in the 1950s with the development of the major tranquilizers. Surgical developments included the heart-lung machine and cardiac catheterization. Mechanical ventilation, introduced in the 1950s, improved resuscitation techniques. Organ transplantation became possible in the 1960s.

Biomedical research continued to be an unquestioned federal budget priority through the 1960s and early 1970s. The government funded important work with recombinant DNA, antiviral compounds, mass production of hormones, and a myriad of other projects. Such investigations had intellectual as well as social and medical consequences. For example, when it became possible to create life outside of the human body, embryos and fetuses came to be thought of in an entirely new light.

These improvements in medical science, as well as the continuing impact of social and environmental factors, had a major impact on U.S. mortality rates and the diseases from which people typically died. Figure 3 summarizes the increases in life expectancy experienced during the twentieth century; and Figure 4, which compares the top ten causes of death in 1900 and 1983,

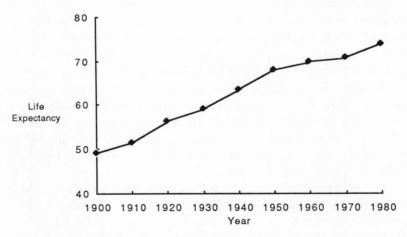

Fig. 3. Life expectancy of Americans at birth, 1900–1980. (Source: National Center for Health Statistics.)

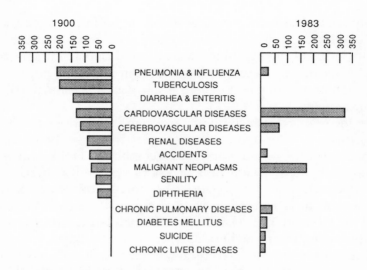

1900   1983

| 350 | 300 | 250 | 200 | 150 | 100 | 50 | 0 | | 0 | 50 | 100 | 150 | 200 | 250 | 300 | 350 |

PNEUMONIA & INFLUENZA
TUBERCULOSIS
DIARRHEA & ENTERITIS
CARDIOVASCULAR DISEASES
CEREBROVASCULAR DISEASES
RENAL DISEASES
ACCIDENTS
MALIGNANT NEOPLASMS
SENILITY
DIPHTHERIA
CHRONIC PULMONARY DISEASES
DIABETES MELLITUS
SUICIDE
CHRONIC LIVER DISEASES

Fig. 4. A comparison of the top ten causes of death among Americans, 1900 and 1983. (Source: National Center for Health Statistics.) Rates represent deaths per 100,000 population.

shows a dramatic shift in causes from infectious diseases to the indirect effects of social problems or lifestyle choices.

Technological expansion during this era affected medical care in many ways. As scientific sophistication increased the complexity of care, clinicians needed more finely honed technical skills. Moreover, the volume of medical knowledge increased exponentially, motivating medical students to specialize as a means of gaining a sense of mastery of the material. Soon specialty care became more lucrative than primary care, with the result that a physician's prestige increasingly became associated with his or her degree of specialization. In 1943 approximately half of all U.S. physicians were general practitioners; by 1978 this figure had fallen to approximately 12 percent.

One effect of the trend toward specialization was to reinforce the drift away from personalized medical care. Where possible, physicians began to substitute a battery of sophisticated tests for the close, hands-on examination made by the general practitioner of earlier years. The notion of medical ethics took clearer shape during this era, being seen by some as a moral counterbalance to the increasing use of technological interventions in medical treatment. And indeed scientific advances increased the number of difficult moral decisions confronting practitioners. In 1958 Pope Pius XII discussed the ethical justifications for removing patients from ventilators. In the mid-1960s it was necessary to formally redefine death in terms of brain function rather than heart and lung function.

The mode of health care delivery also changed during these years. Group practice became much more common; solo practitioners were fewer and house calls rare. A new type of practice arrangement became common in some areas of the country: the prepaid plan. The first large prepaid group practice (PPGP) was started in 1933 by a California physician named Sidney Garfield, who contracted to provide comprehensive medical care for 5,000 men building an aqueduct in return for $1.50 per worker per month from the employer and 5 cents per day from each worker. In 1938 Dr. Garfield contracted with the Kaiser Corporation for prepaid care for the men building the Grand Coulee Dam and their families (10,000 persons in all); and during World War II, Kaiser shipyard workers were also cared for by this plan. Kaiser's experience with this arrangement was so successful that the corporation entered the health care business after the war and eventually enrolled millions, mainly on the West Coast, in its prepaid group practices.

In the 1940s the shortage of physicians surfaced as a health policy issue. One problem was that rural areas and inner cities were inadequately served; another was that primary care physicians were getting harder to find. Yet owing in part to AMA opposition, legislation to increase the number of U.S. physicians was not passed until the early 1960s.

The Health Professions Education Assistance Act of 1963 authorized funds to support the construction of new teaching facilities. Existing medical schools were also given funds for student loans and operating expenses. Additional legislation in 1971 rewarded schools that increased their enrollment. Billions of federal dollars were spent on these growth programs in the 1960s and 1970s. In addition, new laws made it easier for foreign medical graduates to practice; in the early 1970s almost as many foreign as American graduates entered practice in the United States. The training of alternative primary care providers, such as physician assistants and nurse practitioners, was also encouraged. As a result of these manpower policies, the number of physicians in active practice increased by 50 percent between 1960 and 1975.

There was a hospital shortage as well. During the Depression many hospitals had gone bankrupt, and World War II had halted the construction of new facilities. The shortage was particularly acute in rural areas, where many had no access to hospital care. The problem was first addressed by the Hill-Burton Act of 1947, which authorized federal subsidies to states to modernize existing hospitals and construct new ones. In return, hospitals receiving grants had only to provide annual charity care amounting to 2–5 percent of their operating budget. During the next three decades, grants under this law paid for the construction or modernization of 6,500 health care facilities, and the nation's hospital bed capacity approximately doubled.

Modern hospitals bore little resemblance to their predecessors. Research advances and federal money increased their technological sophistication. As religious orders became less a part of the employee force, the missionary aspect of the hospital diminished in importance. And for the first time labor problems surfaced: hospital workers demanded higher wages, and employee strikes led to the unionization of support workers and nurses. Inevitably costs rose. Average daily hospital rates rose from $5 per day in 1940 to $15 per day in 1950, and to more than $200 per day in 1978.

Payment for medical care underwent several changes during this era as well. In 1940 only 9 percent of the population was covered by some form of hospital insurance; eight years later it was 40 percent (Figure 5). Another change was that health insurance premiums came to be paid mainly by employers. Organized labor had become a powerful force during World War II and maintained its strength afterward. Wartime collective bargaining led to the concept of fringe benefits, of which health insurance coverage was (and is) a major component. Many employers agreed to pay the costs of employees' health insurance as part of their wage package.

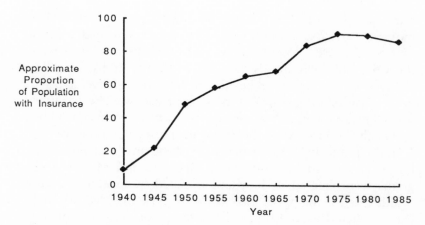

Fig. 5. Proportion of Americans covered by some type of health insurance, 1940–1985. (Sources: Health Insurance Association of America, Blue Cross and Blue Shield Association, Health Care Financing Administration.)

When federal legislation in 1954 exempted employers' payments for health insurance from corporate taxes, employers were effectively encouraged to steer dollars to fringe benefits rather than salary. By 1958 nearly 30 percent of all health insurance enrollees were in collectively negotiated plans.

Things did not work as well for the poor. Certain of payment from the middle and upper classes, which were largely covered by insurance, many hospitals would not admit poor people, or transferred them to second-rate municipal facilities when they were seriously ill. Many impoverished families, particularly in rural areas, had no access to adequate health care. Fifty percent of the aged had no health insurance, and another 25 percent had inadequate coverage.

To the liberal and radical movements of the 1960s this situation was intolerable. A "war on poverty" was declared, and health care was proclaimed to be a citizen's right. Access to care became a prominent social issue, and many believed that public funds should be used to provide medical care of the highest possible quality to the underprivileged.

The Office of Economic Opportunity (OEO) was a government unit developed to lead the so-called war on poverty. When indigent participants in OEO programs were screened, a significant number were found to have untreated diseases. As a result, the OEO allocated funds to projects that would effect "basic changes in the way that health services were delivered to the poor" (Sardell 1983, p. 485). One such project was the Neighborhood Health Center Program, designed to provide comprehensive health services to people living in specific neighborhoods.

In the politically tense atmosphere of the time, the momentum for social reform increased. The Medicare and Medicaid programs were created in 1965 and initiated in 1966 to subsidize health care for the poor, the elderly, and the disabled. Medicare Part A offered federal hospital insurance for persons who were over 65 or permanently disabled; benefits included acute-care hospitalization, limited nursing home care, and other institutional services. Medicare Part B, with the same eligibility as Part A, covered professional fees for medical and surgical services. Medicaid, with a wider range of benefits than Medicare, was developed as a joint federal-state program for the poor.

Concern about access to care for patients with kidney disease led to legislation that further broadened federal responsibility for medical care. In 1973, an End-Stage Renal Disease Program, which pays for transplants or dialysis treatment for beneficiaries, was incorporated into Medicare. End-stage kidney patients are the only group of Medicare beneficiaries who are not required to be either elderly or fully disabled in order to qualify for coverage; their care is subsidized because of their particular disease. Victor Fuchs's 1974 book *Who Shall Live?*, which revealed how hospital committees were choosing patients to receive the limited number of available kidney transplants, reflected societal concerns at that time.

These large-scale government programs, following some thirty years of debate about health care financing, effectively transferred primary responsibility for health care within the public sector from the local to the federal level. With their passage the AMA lost a major battle in its war to maintain full professional independence in health care. Yet despite the initial misgivings of many physicians about Medicare and Medicaid, their benefit to

both patients and providers soon became apparent, and organized medicine came to support them.

In seven decades the U.S. health care industry had been trans-
formed from a prescientific, individualistic cottage industry into
a monolithic, publicly subsidized system. The concern with access to health care and support for its expansion, which had contributed to the creation of this industry, continued for several
years. But serious questions arose about the value of the system,
and in particular about its costs.

*"The price of medical care was already climbing twice as fast as the
cost-of-living index when the Medicare and Medicaid programs went
into operation in mid-1966. The introduction of those programs was
like firing a booster rocket. Physicians' fees, which had been going up
by less than 3 percent annually, began rising more than twice as fast.
The steep climb in hospital charges became even steeper"* (Editors of
Fortune, 1970, p. 19).

One consequence of social reform was the escalation of federal
health care expenditures. Although medical care remained a top
social priority throughout the 1960s and early 1970s, by the mid-
1970s priorities shifted from the creation of new programs to the
maintenance of existing ones. Some were actually dismantled: for
example, Hill-Burton grants were changed to loans in 1970 and
the program was terminated entirely in 1974. Despite these measures, it was estimated that by 1980 the nation had over 100,000
excess beds in acute-care hospitals. Increases in biomedical research spending were also tempered in the late 1960s; until 1968
Congress had always granted the NIH more dollars than were
requested, but in that year only the requested amount was granted
and in later years requested amounts were slashed.

The spiraling costs of health care set the stage for a new movement in the late 1970s: the era of cost control. Part I discusses the
efforts made by the public and private sectors to bring expenditures under rein.

THE ORGANIZATION AND FINANCING OF TODAY'S HEALTH CARE SYSTEM

The current battle follows a decade or two of dreams
and delusions during which both parties to the fray
seem to have believed sincerely that a nation that
defied the law of gravity to go to the moon could also
defy the most fundamental laws of economics.

Uwe Reinhardt

CHAPTER 3

FROM 1979 TO THE PRESENT

Whereas open-ended, largely unbridled budgets for medical care were characteristic of U.S. health policy in the 1960s, by the end of the decade there were already hints of a change in political attitude toward the American health care delivery system. First, the positions of government and other payers underwent subtle change; then society at large became not-so-subtly concerned about health care costs.

The rapid escalation of health care prices in the 1960s and beyond had many causes. General inflation was a major factor; the cost of most goods and services in the economy increased. The health care sector, however, experienced more severe inflation than the rest of the economy. For example, the U.S. Health Care Financing Administration (HCFA) estimated that inflation of physicians' fees *in excess of* general inflation was responsible for 15 percent of the total growth in expenditures for physicians' services from the beginning of the Medicare program to 1984. All of this excess was recorded prior to 1980, when increases slowed to the pace of across-the-board inflation.

Another factor contributing to price increases was greater scientific and technological sophistication, which led to an increase in the complexity of services provided per patient. The same factor increased hospital prices significantly owing to costs associated with the purchase of equipment, the training of specialized employees, and the maintenance of complex machines. Probably the overall effect of technology on the health care sector is mixed: as in other industries, providing a product quicker or better will often decrease its costs. Furthermore, the benefit derived from new technology, in terms of improving the human condition, should not be neglected in assessing its economic effects.

Demographic factors also contributed to the increased costs of health care. Not only did the U.S. population continue to grow, but Medicare and Medicaid subsidies enlarged the patient population by many thousands who previously could not afford care. Moreover, the population is aging. Today well over 10 percent of Americans are over 65, and this proportion is expected to increase substantially in the coming decades. The elderly commonly have chronic diseases that necessitate more hospital admissions, tests, and treatments. On the average, annual medical care for a person over 65 costs more than two and a half times that for a 35-year-old.

In a 1985 publication, HCFA estimated how much several of the above factors contributed to personal health expenditures. From 1965 to 1975, increased intensity of care was a large component of growth in spending. From the mid-1970s through 1984, higher prices were the major cause of increased expenditures. The cumulative effect over time of all factors on hospital costs per day is illustrated in Figure 6. The absolute amounts involved are huge; in 1984 health care became the third-largest United States industry, after food and housing.

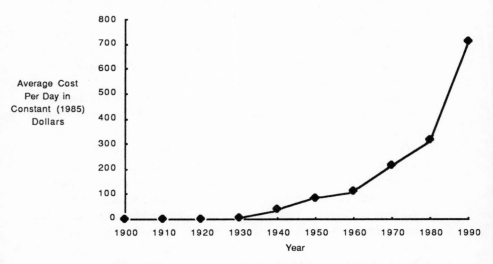

Fig. 6. Average cost of a day in a hospital, 1900–1990. (Sources: Health Insurance Association of America, HCFA, U.S. Government Accounting Office.) A projection is used for 1990.

The Increasing Cost of Health Care

Perhaps more than any other illustration in this book, Figure 7 demonstrates why concerns with the costs of care have profoundly influenced recent health policy. Both as a percentage of gross national product and in actual dollars, health care expenditures began to climb significantly after the Great Society legislation of the 1960s, a trend that continued through the 1970s and into the 1980s. Table 2 presents a series of additional indicators of health care expenditures. Every measure in this table shows a tremendous cost increase over the last two decades.

The sources of dollars spent on current U.S. health care are summarized in Figure 8. In 1965 only 20 percent of health care spending came from public funds. By 1986 the public sector— including local, state, and federal government subsidies and reimbursements—was responsible for over 40 percent of national health expenditures. The private sector, including direct payments from consumers and insurance company reimbursements, accounts for the other 60 percent. Of course, since government

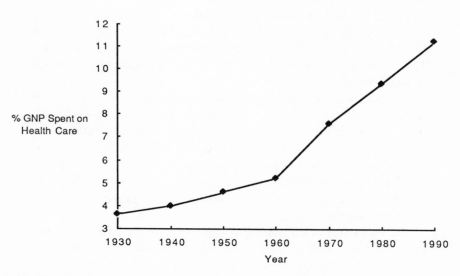

Fig. 7. Percentage of U.S. gross national product spent on health care, 1930–1990. (Source: HCFA.) A projection is used for 1990.

Table 2   **Health Care Expenditures, 1930–1990**

Year	Total U.S. expenditures (billions)	Per capita expenditure	Per capita expenditure in 1985 dollars	Percent change in real per capita expenditure over 5-year period
1930	$3.5	$29	$240	—
1935	2.9	23	176	−27%
1940	4.0	30	225	+28
1945	6.0	55	310	+38
1950	12.7	82	359	+16
1955	17.7	105	413	+15
1960	26.9	146	516	+25
1965	41.9	207	687	+33
1970	75.0	350	952	+39
1975	132.7	591	1,158	+22
1980	248.1	1,054	1,353	+17
1985	422.6	1,710	1,710	+26
1990ᵃ	647.3	2,511	2,353	+38

Sources: HCFA, 1987; Sorkin, 1986.
 ᵃProjection.

revenue derives from taxes, public-sector expenditures are ultimately borne by taxpayers in the private sector.

Figure 8 also presents a breakdown of how today's typical health dollar is spent. Nearly 40 percent goes to hospitals, which for this reason have been targeted first for cost control measures. The proportion now paid from government sources for hospital services is 53 percent.

The Medicare program is the largest health care program in the United States in terms of both expenditures and beneficiaries. In approximately two decades of operation, the program has increased more than thirteenfold, from $4.5 billion to nearly $60 billion, while the number of enrollees has increased by only about one-half, from 20 million to 30 million. As with overall U.S. health care expenditures, the majority of Medicare outlays are spent on hospital care.

The end-stage renal disease component of the Medicare program provides a dismaying example of the effect of a coverage decision on program expenditures. When this benefit was added to the program in the early 1970s it was estimated that expenditures would level off at approximately $200 million annually; the

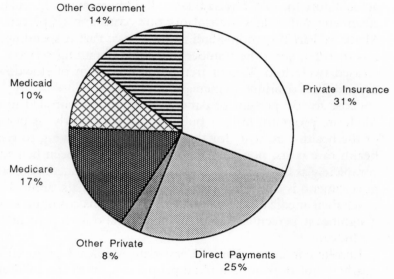

Other Government
14%

Private Insurance
31%

Medicaid
10%

Medicare
17%

Other Private
8%

Direct Payments
25%

Sources

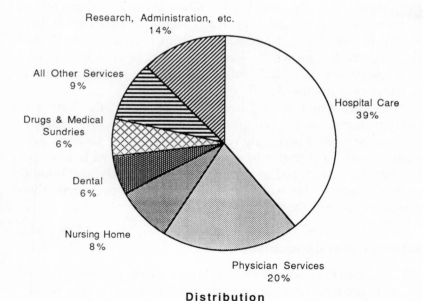

Research, Administration, etc.
14%

All Other Services
9%

Hospital Care
39%

Drugs & Medical
Sundries
6%

Dental
6%

Nursing Home
8%

Physician Services
20%

Distribution

Fig. 8. U.S. health care expenditures, 1986: sources and distribution.
(Source: HCFA.)

actual figure for 1982 was $2 billion. Reimbursements for dialysis treatment and kidney transplants now consume 10 percent of Medicare Part B spending and 1.3 percent of Part A spending. In less than ten years the number of people obtaining services increased twelvefold. Recent trends show no sign of slowdown; expenditures continue to increase.

Close to 100 percent of America's elderly are enrolled in the Medicare program; in 1984 public funds paid nearly 70 percent of the health care costs for those 65 and older. Owing to rising health care costs, however, the elderly have not been helped as completely as Great Society legislators had envisioned. Although government is spending many billions of dollars annually to cover their medical expenses, elderly Americans continue to pay a significant percentage of their income (about 10 percent) for health care.

Enrollment in the joint federal-state Medicaid program has nearly doubled, from 12 million people in 1969 to 21.6 million in 1984. Outlays for Medicaid increased by a factor of eight during this period, to approximately $40 billion annually. Of this total, 17 to 50 percent is paid from state coffers (depending on the wealth of the state), the remainder from federal funds. While the program has grown, so has the number of America's poor. (The effectiveness of Medicaid in covering the health care costs of the poor is discussed in Part II.)

The other major federal health care program, the Veterans Administration system, has grown substantially over the years as well, in the process becoming very costly. In 1985 the Veterans Administration was the third-largest federal agency, with 220,000 full-time employees and an annual budget of $27 billion. Though veterans have traditionally been politically well-protected, this program has been the target of budget cuts in recent years.

International Comparisons

When discussing a society's expenditures on health care, how are we to know how much is enough and how much is too much? One approach to this question is to compare one country's outlays with those of other countries with similar economic systems and similar levels of health status. Table 3 shows spending levels, the availability of health care resources, and statistics on several health markers for the United States and eight other developed countries with free-enterprise industrial economies. *Since all these countries enjoy health indicators that equal, and in most cases exceed, those of the United States and since U.S. expenditures exceed those of all other countries listed, it is at least arguable that "adequate" health care could be provided in this nation at lower cost.*

Political Consensus Develops

In the early 1960s Congress passed legislation supporting generous allocations to the health care sector. But while the federal financial commitment to health care was increasing, the economy was changing for the worse. The Johnson Administration's effort to finance both the Vietnam War and these new domestic programs proved too ambitious and led to severe inflation. The idealism of the Great Society began to fade as budget realities became clearer. Energy and national defense issues became prominent, and health care was no longer a top priority.

Economic troubles continued into the 1970s. The national debt grew alarmingly and productivity slowed, exacerbating the effects of price inflation on the economy. Health care stood out as an area where savings could be made—the more so, critics argued, since sharp increases in health care costs had not brought the expected reductions in morbidity and mortality rates.

By this time, through subsidies for research, medical schools, hospitals, and patient bills, the federal government had long since become the largest single payer of health care costs. It was accordingly the logical candidate to take the lead in reducing costs; and it was soon joined in its efforts by state and private payers.

Such a large and politically powerful industry was not easily brought under legislative control. Political pressure protected many programs from budget cuts; for example, funding for the Hill-Burton program continued until 1974 despite a growing federal concern over an impending hospital bed surplus. There was often lack of agreement on problems and appropriate solutions. Because of the size and decentralization of the U.S. government,

Table 3 **Health and Health Care Characteristics of Nine Industrialized Countries**

Country	Infant mortality, 1982	Expected male longevity at birth, 1980	Health care costs per capita, 1984 U.S. dollars	Health care costs as percent of GNP, 1984	Active MDs per 100,000, 1984	Acute-care hospital beds per 1,000, 1984
U.S.	11.5	70.0	$1,637	11%	210	4.7
Australia	10.0	71.5	984	8	205	—
Canada	9.6	70.2	1,275	8	200	—
Denmark	8.4	71.1	841	6	251	6.1
Finland	6.5	69.5	806	7	220	5.5
Japan	6.6	73.8	818	7	—	—
Sweden	6.8	73.1	1,445	11	252	4.8
U.K.	11.1	70.4	658	6	168	4.0
West Germany	11.6	69.9	1,079	8	230	—

Sources: Fry 1986; National Center for Health Statistics; Schieber 1986.

new policies sometimes worked in opposition to existing policies. Clearly no quick shift in policy was possible.

By the time of the Reagan Administration, however, the political picture was reasonably clear. Federal expenditures had continued to rise: 10 percent of the federal budget was spent on health care by 1984, up from 0.5 percent in 1961. To President Reagan that was high enough, indeed far too high. Reagan brought a free-enterprise philosophy to the presidency. His priorities were lowering taxes, increasing defense spending, and otherwise minimizing government's role in all industries, including health care. The result, in terms of health care policy, is described in later chapters.

Cost-Cutting Efforts by Employers

Employers, too, had their problems with the costs of health care. In 1986 they paid over $90 billion in health care costs on behalf of current and former employees, nearly twice what they had paid in 1980. The higher costs were more than many companies could easily manage.

The inflation of health care prices occurred at a time when U.S. productivity was lagging and many corporations found themselves in fierce competition with foreign manufacturers, particularly the Japanese. Corporate executives examined their operating expenses for ways to cut costs; and only then did most realize the extent to which health care costs were reducing profits. Consider the following examples from the early 1980s:

- $480 of the price of every new car in 1982 paid for health care costs for Chrysler workers. Despite adding many cost control innovations to their benefits program, costs increased to $500 per car in 1984.
- AT&T paid $1.6 billion in medical and dental premiums for workers in 1983.
- The cost of employee health benefits for the Armstrong Tile Company increased 40 percent *each year* from 1978 to 1983.

Findings like these drove more and more employers to look for alternative health insurance arrangements for their employees. (An analogous situation had occurred earlier in the automobile industry; when manufacturers realized that the steel they needed was too expensive and inefficiently produced, they took control of steel production.) New proposals were soon made. Today, *"business people are becoming the most important influence in the re-design of the health care system. They have become the new and potent fourth party. This new party on the scene is pressing for a thorough re-design of the delivery system"* (Freedman 1985, p. 579).

To cease providing employee health insurance might have been a simpler solution, but the tax exemption was a significant advantage for both employer and employee and union opposition to such a move could of course be anticipated. Perhaps the most common strategy adopted by large corporations was self-insurance. Not only can employers lower insurance expenses by assuming the risk themselves, but additional cost savings are achieved because such programs are exempt from most government regulations mandating the extent of coverage. Under this arrangement, which is usually administered by a private insurance company or "third-party administrator," all or most employee claims for medical care are paid out of funds set aside from general operating budgets. This approach has grown in popularity over the years; it is estimated that in 1988 over 50 percent of

U.S. employees with company-sponsored benefits were covered by some form of self-insurance plan.

The Commercial Insurance Industry and Cost Control

Because commercial insurance companies "pass through" any increased health care costs in the form of higher premiums, one might expect such increases not to trouble them. But when premiums got so high that many people elected to risk the occurrence of serious illness and pay their medical expenses out of pocket, the insurance industry became concerned. Another concern was competition from alternative delivery systems such as health maintenance organizations (HMOs), which typically offered expanded health care coverage at equal or lower prices than conventional insurance plans. Still another was the move to self-insurance by many large corporations. Such concerns catalyzed the interest of Blue Cross/Blue Shield in fighting health care price inflation; and the "Blues," who control about half of the private insurance market, led the way for other commercial insurers. As a result, insurance companies joined with corporations and public policymakers in the attempt to limit health care cost increases. These three parties have been called the "new triumvirate" of U.S. health care.

Cost Control and the Surplus of Providers

Figure 9 shows the increase in the number of physicians from 1950 through 1985 and an estimate for the year 2000. The manpower policies of the 1960s and 1970s were so successful that by 1980 the problem had shifted from shortage to surfeit. In that year a blue-ribbon panel—the Graduate Medical Education National Advisory Committee, or GMENAC—forecast not only a significant oversupply of physicians in most surgical and medical subspecialties, but an overall "surplus" of 12 percent by 1990 and 21 percent by 2000. Although estimates vary, many experts believe that the United States already has more practicing physicians than it needs or can afford.

Owing to the surplus of physicians and hospital beds, providers increasingly found themselves competing for patients and dol-

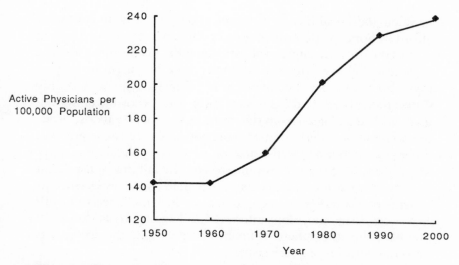

Fig. 9. Number of physicians per 100,000 population, 1950–2000. (Sources: AMA and USDHHS.) Includes both MDs and DOs. Projections are used for 1990 and 2000.

lars. One significant result of this competition was to diminish the political power of the American Medical Association and the American Hospital Association, traditionally two strong opponents of cost control initiatives.

Society Plays a Role

The interests of "society" in containing health care costs vary according to whether one is referring to taxpayers, purchasers of health insurance, or patients. Taxpayers want to pay lower taxes, purchasers lower premiums; patients want the best and most complete health care, which may not be the least expensive. As recently as 1982 the patient's view was the dominant one; in an opinion poll of that year, more than half the people surveyed favored increased government spending on health. As Anderson pointed out, "the American people want choices, easy access, and the latest technology rather than low cost. To the public, the relationship of health services expenditures to the GNP is an abstraction that has no bearing on their daily lives" (1985, p. 23).

Yet as insurance premiums and medical expenses continued to rise, people increasingly saw costs as a problem; they continued to value good health care, but more and more of them could not afford it. Some 68 percent of those polled in a 1985 survey named cost as the greatest single problem facing the health care industry.

As noted above, this new emphasis arose in part from misgivings about whether the money was being well spent. U.S. life expectancy, which had been increasing since record-keeping began, reached a plateau from the mid-1950s to the late 1960s, "leading some to wonder whether more medical care made any real difference in human well-being or survival" (Blendon 1983, p. 1880). Also, as it became popular to cite the failures of the Great Society (such as increased costs) rather than its successes (such as benefits to the indigent), people became less interested in health as a social issue and more interested in keeping costs down. In the 1980s the atmosphere of financial crisis made the arguments for cost control more persuasive.

The media drove the message home with references to the health care cost "crisis." Soon the average American was very aware of the problem, and for the first time society in the aggregate sought to slow the growth of the health care sector instead of offering *carte blanche* for expansion.

The tides of support for health care had begun to shift in the 1970s, but the true era of cost control dates from the early 1980s. The following quotation captures the spirit of the new era:

Although there is no magic formula for determining a precise limit on what a country can afford to spend for health care, there is a limit. Every dollar spent on health care is a dollar that cannot be spent on something else. No set of expenditures can rise faster than the gross national product forever. At some point, health-care expenditures must slow down to the rate of growth of the gross national product" (Thurow, 1984, p. 1569).

As part of this process, the major payers have begun to gain control of the health care sector. Health care financing and organization are evolving within the constraints set by these payers. Cost control measures by government (as both payer and regulator), the business sector, and the health insurance industry are examined in the following chapters.

CHAPTER 4

HEALTH CARE AS A MARKET COMMODITY

At this point, a brief digression into basic economic theory is necessary, since cost containment interventions are based on this theory. As we shall see, the market for health care is replete with economic anomalies when compared to other consumer markets. The differences between health care and other markets help explain why some cost containment measures are effective while others fail.

The Balance of Supply and Demand

Supply-demand theory is used by economists to describe the relationship between the price of a product and the quantity purchased of that product. Health care services are products. Those who offer the product, such as hospitals and physicians, are its producers. Those who purchase it, including patients, government, and insurance companies, are its consumers.

Consumer demand for a given product depends on several factors, among them the price of the product, the prices of goods or services that could be substituted for it, consumer income, and consumer tastes or preferences. Other factors may also affect demand, such as third-party insurance coverage, which decreases the price paid by the consumer. The quantity (Q) of a product that producers offer is its supply (S). Supply, like demand (D), is generally responsive to price (P): the higher the price, the greater the quantity supplied. The price of the product goes up as demand increases. The inverse also occurs: if demand decreases, the price will fall in response, which in turn leads to reduced supply.

A demand curve, such as Figure 10, graphically illustrates the theoretical relationship between price and demand for medical services. This simplified model suggests that consumers will demand more visits to physicians as the price per visit decreases, and suppliers (physicians) will charge more per visit as the demand increases. In theory, the intersection of the supply and demand lines reflects the equilibrium where the P and Q of the product are determined.

These classic supply-demand relationships do apply for some health care products. For example, many optometrists and ophthalmologists offer competitive rates for eye examinations and glasses, knowing that prospective patients might compare prices before choosing a provider. Many (if not most) health care products, however, are not governed by simple laws of supply and demand. Some problems in applying supply-demand theory to health care are outlined below.

The Uniqueness of Health Care

Classic economic theories base their assumptions on the consistent nature of the supplied product. But health care is heterogeneous, in essence tailor-made for each patient depending on the illness and on decisions made during the patient-provider encounter. A medical service may be fairly well circumscribed, such as suturing a laceration; but just as often the product is nebulous,

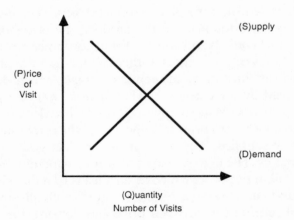

Fig. 10. An economic model of the market for physician services.

such as spending an hour reassuring a healthy but anxious patient that an imagined brain tumor is nonexistent. The differing nature of these services must be quantified if they are to conform to supply-demand theory.

The Inefficient Allocation of Health Care

Classic theory suggests that demand for a product is based on consumers' willingness and ability to pay for it. However, patients who need medical care may be unable to purchase it, or providers may not be available to "produce" it. Moreover, medical care is a uniquely valuable product: it directly affects the quality of a person's life, and at the extreme can mean the difference between life and death. In the case of health care we must expand the strict sense of demand to include *need* for the product. From an ethical perspective, many believe that health care should be delivered on the basis of need, not ability to pay.

Another consideration making supply-demand analysis difficult is the value that society in the aggregate derives from the health of its individual members. This is termed an "external effect," since it affects neither the consumer who purchases the service nor the provider who supplies it. The classic example of a medical service with an external effect is vaccination. The benefit obtained by the patient from the service is less than the benefit enjoyed by society as a whole when its members are vaccinated. Thus if some people are unable or unwilling to pay for vaccinations, the product is supplied anyway and the public sector picks up the bill.

Consumer Dependency

The supply-demand model also assumes a knowledgeable buyer, a doubtful assumption when it comes to health care because patients often do not know what kind of care they need. The need may be obvious enough in the case of pain, bleeding, or impaired function, but just as often it is subtle or hidden. Furthermore, emotional needs and other personal characteristics can affect the need for care, leading patients to demand more or less care than their physical condition necessitates.

When changes in the price of a product lead to changes in demand for that product, the product is said to be price-elastic. Some types of medical services are price-elastic, but many are not. The classic case of price inelasticity in health care is the life-or-death situation. An unconscious trauma victim arrives at the hospital in an ambulance: medical care is provided on the assumption that the patient, if awake, would request it regardless of its price.

Another cause of price inelasticity in the health care market is the low degree of product interchangeability. If steak costs too much, we can buy hamburger instead. But if a patient needs an appendectomy, what can be substituted to achieve a benefit comparable to the surgical procedure?

The Creation of Demand by Providers

Another significant exception to classical economic theory is that the health care industry can to some extent create demand for its own product (for example, by scheduling a return appointment or recommending surgery). This ability on the supplier's part complicates the relationships between supply and demand, and between supply and price.

It also raises an important ethical question: to what extent are patients helped by physician-initiated medical care, and to what extent is the initiation in the practitioner's self-interest? According to Wilensky, "Physician initiation is inducement only when services are recommended above and beyond what the patient would be willing to pay for if the patient knew as much as the physician" (1983, p. 259). The difference between initiation and inducement is subtle but critical. Initiation is appropriate, inducement a violation of professional ethics.

Ethical considerations apart, however, the health care consumer is largely dependent on the producer for information concerning his or her condition and possible treatment, and is heavily influenced by the producer's recommendations. The producer in effect acts as the consumer's agent in purchasing medical services, which makes the relationship between doctor and patient very unlike the usual producer-consumer relationship.

This control of demand by providers is one reason why the

dramatic increase in the number of hospitals and physicians has not led to price wars among them. During the 1970s an increase in the supply of physicians occurred simultaneously with increasing prices and higher demand for medical services. In several studies the number of practitioners in a given area has been found to correlate directly with both health care prices and the quantity of services provided. For example, the number of certain surgical procedures performed in a community was shown to be correlated with the number of surgeons there, and not necessarily with the incidence of surgically correctable disease. However, not all researchers are in agreement on what these studies mean. Some believe that physician inducement is a relatively minor factor in consumers' decisions to use medical services.

On a related theme, Milton Roemer, a physician and health policy researcher, has found a direct correlation between the number of hospital beds in a given area and the use of those beds, when all other variables likely to affect their use were held constant. "Roemer's Law" accordingly states that hospital beds will fill up to the extent that they are available; in effect, "the supply of beds creates a demand for those beds" (Feldstein 1983, p. 89).

Barriers to Competition

A prerequisite to the application of supply-demand theory is that competition exist among suppliers of the same product. According to the theory, as more products are provided, production improves and per-unit cost decreases. In general, however, this is not true of appendectomies, or even annual check-ups. The one-on-one nature of most health care products is a key reason why health care providers have had a difficult time competing primarily on the basis of price.

Also, of course, "the unpredictable and acute nature of many health problems often precludes 'shopping' for health services. A person afflicted by life-threatening symptoms is hardly in a position to search the market for the 'best deal'" (Hsiao 1979, p. 23).

Another factor affecting competition is the relative lack of competitive pricing for professional fees. Historically, practitioners set their own fees without regard to those of other practitioners; they charged what they thought fair or what the market would bear. In later years, as we shall see in Chapter 6, complex third-party price-setting mechanisms allowed for such practices and thus in effect supported them.

Norms of behavior have also contributed to independent fee-setting: it was long considered unprofessional not only to disparage another practitioner's services or fees but to advertise one's own. For many years the codes of professional ethics of the AMA and other professional associations prohibited advertising. As we shall see, the prohibition is now illegal, but the reluctance to advertise is still widespread. One result is that it is hard for a consumer to base a decision on price.

When medical care prices did not decrease in the 1970s despite an increasing number of active physicians and hospital beds, it became clear that a simple competitive model was not adequate to describe the health care market. As Alain Enthoven, a health economist, notes, physicians acted in various ways to suppress competition: among other things, they obstructed the use of prepaid group plans and other lower-cost providers, refused to grant hospital privileges to practitioners who discounted their fees, and boycotted insurance companies that put a ceiling on reimbursement rates. Thanks in part to an active and well-funded lobby in Washington, they were generally successful in keeping prices high.

It is the goal of antitrust legislation to prevent such behavior and to promote competition. The medical profession was exempt from antitrust regulation until 1975, when the Supreme Court upheld a lower court's ruling that the Virginia state bar association could not establish or enforce a minimum fee schedule for lawyers. By treating the legal profession like other trades, the court decision paved the way for the medical profession to be considered a "trade" as well.

The Federal Trade Commission then successfully sued the AMA to remove its prohibition on advertising. Physicians and hospitals may now advertise their services, and many do. Indeed, marketing efforts have become an important aspect of profitable private practice management in the 1980s. Unfortunately, however, antitrust legislation has adversely affected the medical profession's ability to regulate itself, since any attempt to impose internal standards—whether planning medical school class sizes, regulating peer behavior, or policing state licensing criteria— may lead to an allegation of antitrust activity.

Although competition is not applicable to every aspect of medical care, it is a realistic possibility in some sectors of the health care industry, such as shopping for health insurance. In 1978 Enthoven submitted a plan to the Carter Administration that was based on competition between alternative insurance packages. His "Consumer-Choice Health Plan" would have given tax credits or vouchers to taxpayers and direct subsidies to low-income citizens. The voucher amount would have been adequate to purchase a basic health care package; taxpayers could choose their own plan, supplementing the voucher with their own funds if they wanted more expensive coverage.

The proposal was designed to induce insurers to offer less expensive and more comprehensive health plans. Only a few aspects of the plan would have been federally mandated, notably an annual period of open enrollment and a limit on out-of-pocket expenses per family. Otherwise insurers would have been free to compete for enrollees, using any benefit structure the market would bear.

Although the Enthoven plan was not in the end adopted, it prompted much discussion of the role of competition in the health care sector. Since 1978 payers and policymakers have initiated a wide variety of cost-controlling approaches—some old, some new, some based on market regulation, others on increasing market competition, but all designed to correct one or more of the market imperfections discussed in this chapter. These measures are explored in the following chapters.

CHAPTER 5

COSTS: THE CONSUMER'S PERSPECTIVE

Medical bills are expensive; a hospital stay of moderate length can easily cost more than a new automobile. Moreover, people become ill unpredictably, making it desirable to pool risks with others. For these and other reasons, a large majority of Americans now have health insurance. The structure and availability of this third-party coverage have had a profound impact on the United States health care system.

The Health Insurance Benefit Structure

Approximately 85 percent of all Americans have some type of insurance coverage for health care. Approximately 55 percent of all families are insured by private insurers such as Blue Cross/Blue Shield and the so-called commercial companies, 10 percent by health maintenance organizations (HMOs) or other prepaid plans, and 21 percent by government-sponsored programs. The rest, about 15 percent, lack insurance coverage of any kind.

Most private "indemnity"* insurance policies cover hospitalization and its associated professional fees; typical additional benefits include diagnostic services such as laboratory tests and x-rays. Additionally, a "major medical" policy is often purchased, covering services excluded from the core policy, such as office visits to physicians and the portion of hospital bills exceeding a predetermined limit (say, $50,000). Conventional insurance programs rarely cover any care not directly related to an illness; preventive services are usually excluded for this reason. Also most

---

*Conventional insurance programs are considered *indemnity* programs because the insurer agrees to protect the beneficiary against a liability, namely, what he or she will have to pay for medical care.

policies do not cover long-term chronic care, such as provided by nursing homes, for any extended period.

Insurance premiums are priced according to "actuarial risk," a complicated calculation based on statistics of various kinds of illness incurred in various age/sex groups. The insurer's risk is more predictable, and premiums are accordingly lower, when expenses are dispersed among a large number of enrollees. For this reason, and because an insurance company's administrative overhead is lower when it deals with a single company employing about 1,000 people than when it deals with 1,000 people individually, a person purchasing "individual" health insurance outside of an employer-sponsored "group" must usually accept either prohibitively expensive premiums or limited coverage.

Although fixed premium prices assure a degree of predictability in health care costs, most policies require the policyholder to pay a portion of the costs of care when such costs are in fact incurred. Insurance companies favor such arrangements not only because they reduce the company's payout, but because the patient's liability may make him or her think twice about seeking medical care not really needed.

Cost-sharing provisions may take a variety of forms. One is co-insurance, in which the policyholder pays a predetermined percentage of the medical bill: thus a 20 percent co-insurance rate means that the patient pays 20 percent of the total charge. Another is co-payment, in which the policyholder pays a fixed dollar amount per unit of service: for example, $5 per visit toward whatever the physician charges. Still another is a deductible arrangement, in which the patient pays the deductible amount (say, $100) out of pocket before any insurance benefits are paid. Most policies have an upper limit on cost-sharing, known as a "stoploss." Beyond this point the insurance will cover all expenses, usually up to a maximum coverage amount (say, $1 million).

These arrangements frequently occur in combination. For example, a patient receives his or her first medical bill of the year, totaling $400. The services received are covered by an insurance policy, which stipulates an annual deductible of $100 with a 20 percent co-insurance rate thereafter. The patient is therefore responsible for paying $100 plus 20 percent of the remaining $300, or a total of $160. The insurance company pays $240. If the next bill in the same year is $200, the patient pays only the co-insurance of $40 and the insurance company pays the rest.

The nonprofit Blue Cross/Blue Shield companies are different from profit-making private insurance companies. One difference can be linked to the early role that hospitals played in developing such insurance plans; the Blues have not traditionally required co-insurance or deductible payments for inpatient care, and their policyholders accordingly pay higher premiums. Second, although these companies do their best to make sure that revenues exceed expenses, all excess revenue is reinvested in the company, not paid out to shareholders. This and certain tax advantages help to keep their premiums competitive with plans making greater use of cost-sharing, and to maintain their market share (about half of the private insurance business).

Medicare and Medicaid are the public sector's insurance programs. Medicare Part A is supported by a trust fund that is replenished annually by Social Security payroll taxes paid by both employers and employees. Eligible enrollees pay no premiums for Part A, but are required to pay a significant deductible as well as co-insurance. Approximately 25 percent of Medicare Part B, which is considered a supplemental insurance program, is funded by enrollee premiums, with the remainder coming from general federal funds. Part B requires a monthly premium and incorporates co-insurance as well as an annual deductible.

Medicaid is considered "assurance," not "insurance," because eligibles receive coverage without paying into the program. It is funded entirely from public sources: about half by federal funds, and half by state and local funds. This ratio varies from state to state, with the federal share higher in poorer states. Medicaid eligibles pay no premiums or co-insurance, although some states require a small co-payment for prescription drugs and other services.

Nearly every citizen over age 65 is enrolled in Medicare Part A, and more than 90 percent are also enrolled in Part B. By contrast, less than half of the nation's poor, who constitute some 13 percent of the population, are covered by the Medicaid program.*

---

* In 1985, the poverty level for a family of four was defined as an annual income of $11,000 or less. The average income of U.S. families of two or more persons was $30,000.

Medicare Part A is in financial trouble. Payouts from its trust fund have so far exceeded revenue that according to one projection there will be no funds left by 1989 and a $100 billion deficit by 1995. Since current federal law prohibits using general revenue sources to subsidize the program, other ways must be found to deal with the problem; some possibilities are described below. Medicare Part B and Medicaid are in better shape, backed as they are by general revenues, but policymakers are understandably intent on controlling outlays for these programs as well. Table 4 shows the tremendous growth experienced by Medicare Part B over time.

Table 4   **Medicare Part B Enrollment, Reimbursement Amounts, and Claims Volume, 1967–1984**
(columns 2–4 in millions)

Fiscal year	Number of beneficiaries	Total dollars	Number of claims	Claims per beneficiary
1967	17.8	$664	19.7	1.1
1968	18.0	1,390	34.2	1.9
1969	18.8	1,645	39.3	2.1
1970	19.3	1,979	43.8	2.3
1971	19.7	2,035	49.1	2.5
1972	20.0	2,255	54.5	2.7
1973	20.4	2,391	58.5	2.9
1974	22.6	2,874	68.0	3.0
1975	23.3	3,765	81.4	3.5
1976	24.1	4,672	93.5	3.9
1977	24.8	5,867	110.0	4.4
1978	25.6	6,852	122.1	4.8
1979	26.3	8,259	136.2	5.2
1980	26.9	10,144	154.5	5.7
1981	27.5	12,345	171.1	6.2
1982	28.0	14,806	188.3	6.7
1983	28.5	17,487	208.4	7.3
1984	29.0	19,473	229.0	7.9

Source: U.S. Congress 1986, p. 41.

Capitation Payment Methods

Some indemnity insurance plans reimburse the beneficiary for covered services paid for out of pocket; others directly reimburse the provider on the consumer's behalf. Almost all such plans pay the provider on a fee-for-service basis *after* the care has been delivered. But a very different arrangement, still relatively uncommon in the United States, is growing in importance. Under this scheme, known as capitation, health care providers are paid in advance on a per capita basis for patients committed to using their services.

Such an arrangement usually occurs only within nontraditional delivery settings such as health maintenance organizations. Therefore, from a provider's perspective, capitation is often viewed more as an organizational arrangement than as an insurance program. From the patient's perspective, however, capitation *is* an insurance mechanism. Like conventional insurance, capitation protects patients against financial loss from illness; and of course the prepayment is analogous to purchasing an insurance premium. Capitation also has important effects on the health care delivery process, since under capitation schemes patients are generally restricted to those providers who participate in the program.

In a capitation plan, enrollees or their employers pay a predetermined fee for a year of coverage. Coverage is typically comprehensive, including preventive care (such as well-child checkups), office visits, prescription drugs, and hospital care as necessary. Capitation plans rarely, if ever, require deductibles or cost-sharing, but small co-payments on the order of $5 may be required for some services. The predominant form of capitation arrangement, the health maintenance organization or HMO, is discussed in Chapter 6.

Effects of Insurance Coverage

Most insurance, including fire, theft, and life, is against unexpected occurrences. Health insurance differs in that most people expect to need medical services. Whereas the only way a policyholder can act to get a return on his investment in fire or life insurance is by arson or suicide, both of which negate all coverage, it is to the consumer's economic advantage to seek a return on his or her health insurance by obtaining health care: by getting, as it were, what was paid for. This has been called the "more-is-better" incentive of health insurance.

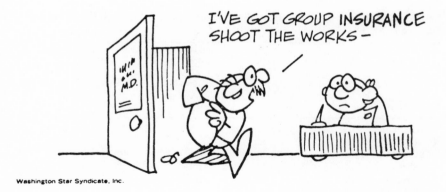

I'VE GOT GROUP INSURANCE SHOOT THE WORKS—

Washington Star Syndicate, Inc.

More-is-better incentives are particularly compelling for enrollees with first-dollar coverage, that is, where there is no up-front cost-sharing. Since most capitation plans are essentially of this sort, some providers in capitation systems attempt to limit the more-is-better tendency by lengthening the waiting time for nonemergency appointments or placing other nonmonetary barriers before the patient. The tendency to use and perhaps overuse a health insurance policy because of the strong financial incentive to do so has been labeled by economists the "moral hazard" phenomenon.

In 1986 employers paid more than 70 percent of the $141 billion annually spent on non-government-sponsored health insurance, or some 22 percent of all health care expenditures. Government paid an additional 41 percent of the nation's health care bill, and patients paid 25 percent of the total out of pocket and another 10 percent as private insurance premiums. The out-of-pocket percentage has decreased sharply over the last several decades; as a result, direct costs to patients have remained fairly constant. Table 5 presents some detailed information on typical consumer uses and costs of different types of services in 1986.

Effects of Cost-Sharing on Demand

The nature and extent of cost-sharing provisions in an insurance policy influences the consumer's demand for services. For example, the purchase of a policy with a typical 20 percent co-insurance provision results in an 80 percent decrease in the pa-

Table 5 **Statistics on Medical Services Use and Costs by Type of Service, 1986**

Type of medical service	Estimated use per year per person	Approximate percentage of popula- tion receiv- ing services in year	Typical cost per unit of service	Approximate percentage of all costs borne di- rectly by individuals	Approximate percentage of U.S. health care costs
Hospital admission	0.11	10%	$4,550	10%	39%
Physician services					
Ambulatory visit	5.00	75	40	50	12
Surgery	0.20	15	600	20	5
In-hospital visit	0.60	10	30	20	3
Medication/drugs[a]	4.30	60	15	70	4
Dental visit	1.80	50	30	70	6
Nursing home admission	0.05	0.5	25,000[b]	50	8

Sources: USDHHS, NCHSR 1987; HCFA 1987; USDHHS 1987; AMA 1986; USDHHS, NCHSR 1982.
  [a]Prescribed out of hospital.
  [b]Cost per year.

tient's out-of-pocket cost when medical services are obtained. A substantial increase in providers' charges must take place before patients with such coverage experience significant increases in their medical bills. This insulation from actual costs has two important effects: it permits inflation in health care prices to occur more easily, and it increases the use of services by policyholders.

The Health Insurance Experiment was an extensive federally financed study conducted by the Rand Corporation from 1974 to 1982. Some 2,000 families living in six cities were randomly assigned to one or another of fourteen insurance plans with four degrees of cost-sharing, ranging from 0 to 95 percent. For the three plans with some degree of cost-sharing, differing upper limits were set on annual out-of-pocket expenditures, ranging from 5 to 15 percent of income to a maximum of $1,000. The study found that members of families with lower cost-sharing percentages visited physicians more frequently and entered the hospital more often than members of families with higher percentages. The study's findings are summarized in Table 6. On the basis of this study and others, one expert concluded that a typical insurance policy approximately doubles the demand for services.

A major objective of health insurance executives is to set com-

Table 6 **Annual Health Care Expenses per Person by Level of Co-insurance, 1974—1978**
(1974—1978 current dollar averages across four sites)

Coinsurance paid by consumer (percent)	Total expenditure	Ambulatory expenditure
0 (free care)	$401	$186
25[a]	346	149
50[a]	328	120
95[b]	254	114

Source: Rand Health Insurance Experiment. (For more complete results, including confidence intervals, see Newhouse 1981.)
[a]With a family stop-loss of $1,000.
[b]Family pays 95 percent up to $450 deductible.

petitively priced premiums that will cover all services supplied to enrollees while leaving some surplus as a return to investors. Thus their concern is to forecast, and if possible decrease, enrollees' use of health care services. Government policymakers, who are also major insurers thanks to public-sector programs, have the same goals. As the End-Stage Renal Disease Program has demonstrated, coverage decisions have important budgetary consequences.

Cutting Costs by Cost-Sharing

To most people the workings of third-party payers take place in the proverbial "black box." Consumers pay insurance premiums or taxes into the box, and coverage emerges. Practitioners submit claims forms for services provided, and the box provides reimbursements (usually). The dynamic environment in which the black box operates has been largely ignored. This ignorance is understandable enough, since until recently U.S. health care policy has been characterized by the expansion of benefits to providers and patients; but like most kinds of ignorance it has had its costs.

When consumers bear some responsibility for health care costs, the inflationary effects of the moral hazard phenomenon are diminished. A variety of efforts to control costs by decreasing people's incentives to use health care services have been made by government, private insurers, and employers. In particular, two methods have been used to pare down the insulation between patients and their bills: providing fewer benefits at the same premium price, and increasing required payments for co-insurance, deductibles, and the like. The first approach places consumers directly at risk for a service. The second raises their threshold for seeking care for covered services, and also decreases the payer's outlays.

The public sector has made extensive use of cost-sharing to keep costs down. HCFA has regularly increased the deductible that must be paid by Medicare Part A beneficiaries before their coverage is activated. A single deductible is paid for all hospital services used during a defined benefit period. A new benefit period begins when the patient has been out of the hospital for sixty days. The deductible has gone up every year since the inception of the Medicare program; in 1987 it was $492.

For Medicare Part B, the monthly premium was originally designed to pay half the program costs; federal funds were to pay the other half. Today federal funds pay 75 percent of costs and premium revenues only 25 percent, despite repeated increases in premium charges and deductibles. In 1987 the premium was $17.90 monthly, with an annual deductible of $75 and 20 percent co-insurance; and for 1988 the premium was increased by 38.5 percent, to $24.80, to cover increased expenditures. As a result of price inflation and these cost-sharing approaches, "Older persons now pay a larger portion of their income for health care than they did before Medicare was enacted" (Blumenthal 1986, p. 722).

The intended disincentive effect of Medicare cost-sharing is undercut to some degree by additional insurance coverage available to most beneficiaries and by the Medicaid program, which pays co-insurance and deductibles for indigent Medicare enrollees. Some 60 percent of Medicare enrollees purchase supplemental private insurance (often termed "medi-gap" insurance) to pay Medicare deductibles and co-insurance charges. In effect, most Medicare beneficiaries have not found cost-sharing a significant disincentive to overuse of the program.

One way the public sector could cut its health care expenditures is by eliminating tax exemptions on health insurance premiums. Billions of dollars in potential federal and state revenues are lost each year from these exemptions: approximately $26 billion in 1983. Although Congress has threatened several times to impose a tax on employers' contributions to benefit packages, intense lobbying has successfully blocked such action. In 1982 the amount of tax-deductible personal medical care expenses (which include contributions toward premiums) was reduced, but employers' deductions were preserved.

In the private sector, commercial insurance companies have always relied on cost-sharing, and this approach remains standard. Even the Blues, which traditionally had more limited cost-sharing provisions, have recently introduced a "Partnership Program" that incorporates significant deductibles (as high as $500) and co-insurance.

Employer plans increasingly incorporate employee co-payments. Some plans offer employees more expensive and less expensive options; those who choose the more costly policy must pay the difference in premium costs out of pocket. Others limit employees' choice of physicians to so-called preferred providers who charge less. (Preferred provider plans are discussed in Chapter 6.) Deductibles have increased for corporate employees as well: a 1984 survey of 1,200 companies found that 52 percent had deductibles, up from 17 percent in 1982. Also in 1982 some 75 percent of surveyed companies provided full hospital room and board coverage; only a year later, in 1983, that figure had fallen to 50 percent.

Employers have come up with several innovative plans that indirectly involve cost-sharing. One such plan offers each employee minimal coverage—for example, only hospitalization coverage—plus a special account containing additional funds for medical services not covered by the policy. If the employee uses such services, the bills are paid from that account. At the end of the year, a portion of any unused money in the account is returned to the employee as a bonus. This gives the employee a direct incentive to minimize the use of medical care.

Many businesses have started occupational health clinics, health promotion programs, or "employee assistance programs" that treat substance abuse. Employers expect these programs to result in healthier, happier employees who will require less medical care.

Consumer-Oriented Controls

In addition to cost-sharing provisions, many insurers offer programs designed to decrease the use of specific kinds of services. One example is the second-surgical-opinion program. If a surgical procedure is advised, the program pays for consultation with a second surgeon. If the two surgeons disagree, the program will pay for yet a third consultation. Some insurers (or employers) require a beneficiary to obtain a second opinion before undergoing any major elective procedure; others simply offer the second opinion as an option. An estimated 20 percent of all patients in such programs eventually do not undergo the surgery initially recommended. Of Fortune 500 companies, 82 percent have such programs.

Because outpatient procedures are less expensive than the same services provided in a hospital, some payers have introduced programs to encourage the use of outpatient facilities. For example, in 1982 Medicare elected to pay 100 percent of the physician's fee for ambulatory surgery but only 80 percent for inpatient surgery, thus creating a strong incentive for patients to use outpatient facilities when possible. Also in 1982 Medicare issued a list of procedures that would be reimbursed *only* on an outpatient basis barring special contraindications.

Many large corporations now hire nonphysician reviewers (sometimes known as "case managers") to monitor the use of major services such as elective hospital admissions or rehabilitation therapy. Their purpose is to see that the corporation gets its money's worth. "Corporations and insurers are quick to point out that they never tell an employee not to have a hysterectomy or forbid anyone from entering the hospital to see if that lesion is cancerous. All they do is, at times, decline to pick up the full bill for a procedure they deem unnecessary. The patient, they insist, can do as he pleases" (Kleinfield 1986, p. F3).

An alternative system, usually known as the "gatekeeper" system, is used by some private insurance and state Medicaid plans to cut down on the duplication of services and on unnecessary referrals. In this system a primary-care physician is appointed to act as care coordinator for the beneficiary. The patient must call the gatekeeper before any nonemergency care is received from other providers, or services will not be reimbursed. For a monthly payment in addition to any fee-for-service reimbursements, the gatekeeper provides whatever coordinating activities are needed.

It has proved difficult to recruit physicians to serve as gatekeepers, especially in Medicaid programs, where low monthly payments (sometimes as low as $3) are clearly inadequate compensation for the physician's time and trouble. Many plans, however, have incorporated this approach, notably HMOs.

Government Retrenchments

The Reagan Administration, as part of its effort to decrease government spending wherever possible, took several steps to reduce federal involvement in health care. The Neighborhood Health Center Program was phased out; though since then, direct "Community Health Center" funding to about 600 free-standing clinics has been reinstated. The National Health Service Corps, which subsidized the medical education of providers willing to practice in underserved areas, was all but eliminated. The Veterans Administration hospital system was also targeted for further budget cuts.

With regard to the Medicare and Medicaid programs, the Reagan Administration sought to decrease both the number of enrollees and the number of reimbursable services. One proposal was to raise the age of eligibility. "Since Medicare began, life expectancy for those reaching 65 years of age has increased by 2 years for women and one year for men. Increased longevity has provided a rationale for proposals to advance the age of eligibility for Medicare" (Aiken 1984, p. 1198). This idea found some support in 1985, when Congress increased the age of eligibility for full Social Security retirement benefits from 65 to 67 commencing in the year 2000, but the age of eligibility for Medicare benefits has not yet been raised.

At the state level, Medicaid expenditures were reduced by decreasing the income level above which families do not qualify for

Medicaid, decreasing the income level at which a family is considered "medically indigent,"* and reducing the number of services covered (within the limits set by federal guidelines).

Studies have shown capitation plans to be less expensive than other types of insurance, in part because of financial incentives to the practitioner. Total costs, including premium payments plus out-of-pocket expenses, average 10 to 40 percent lower for HMO enrollees than for beneficiary groups with comparable health status covered under conventional indemnity insurance plans. Given these figures, the Reagan Administration understandably encouraged Medicare beneficiaries to enroll in Medicare HMOs and "competitive medical plans" (CMPs), which are primarily HMOs that are not "federally qualified" by HCFA's Office of Pre-paid Health Care. Such plans offer members a "richer benefit package and more predictable out-of-pocket costs, but their freedom of choice of providers is restricted to the physicians and hospitals of the health plan in which a person enrolls" (Ellwood 1986, p. 183).

Medicare HMOs are known as "risk-contract" HMOs because they are under government contract to provide care for a fixed amount equal to 95 percent of the average costs of all care received by similar Medicare beneficiaries in the geographic area covered by the plan. Plans are also allowed to charge premiums, which have ranged from zero to more than $38 monthly. Alternative plans offer services not available to Medicare beneficiaries in the traditional system, including extended hospital days, preventive care, drugs, eye care, dental care, and expanded mental health benefits. After a predetermined profit any savings that such HMOs realize above the federal reimbursement level must be passed along to enrollees in the form of increased benefits.

Promotion efforts have greatly increased the enrollment of Medicare beneficiaries in HMOs. As of 1987 over 900,000 beneficiaries, or 3.0 percent of the Medicare population, were enrolled in about 150 such plans. Surveys of Medicare enrollees have shown them to be satisfied with HMO care. In mid-1987, how-

---

*Families with incomes above the cutoff level for Medicaid coverage but with sufficiently large medical expenses are termed "medically indigent" and are eligible for Medicaid.

ever, after a handful of plans were found to be offering poor-quality care, federally funded Peer Review Organizations (which were previously established to monitor Medicare-supported hospital care) began monitoring risk-contract HMOs.

Summation: The Consumer and Cost Controls

Theoretically, patients required to pay more for their care will seek less of it, and practitioners in turn will provide fewer services. Yet increased patient cost-sharing has had only a moderate effect on medical costs, particularly hospital costs. Results from the Rand Study confirm that consumers are less responsive to cost-sharing for acute-care hospital services than for ambulatory services, probably because it is the physician, not the consumer, who usually makes the decision to hospitalize. "While individuals may choose their physicians, doctors usually determine the kind and quantity of health services individuals consume. While doctors may have some knowledge of the individual's financial resources, there is little evidence that these considerations have much influence on the type of care prescribed" (Sorkin 1975, p. 23).

Apart from ethical considerations, it should be emphasized that whereas increased cost-sharing can decrease a patient's use of medical care, it can also decrease his or her access to needed care. This could potentially lead to the identification and treatment of diseases at later stages, which may be more expensive in the long run.

Consumer-focused cost controls can and do help to reduce costs, but for all these reasons there are clear limits to how much they can accomplish. As the next chapters demonstrate, third-party payers have accordingly chosen to focus most of their cost-control efforts on the providers of care.

CHAPTER 6

COSTS: THE PROVIDER'S PERSPECTIVE

Overall, physicians receive approximately 60 percent of their revenue from insurance programs and 40 percent directly from patients. The percentages vary according to specialty, location, and other factors. For example, insurers have traditionally reimbursed *procedures* at higher rates than *cognitive services* such as physical or psychiatric examinations. (Most specialists' services are predominantly in one or the other of these categories.) Surgeons receive a much greater percentage of their income from third-party insurance companies than pediatricians, psychiatrists, and other physicians who offer most of their services in an office setting. These coverage differences are believed to be largely responsible for income differences among specialties. For example, in 1985 United States surgeons earned an average taxable income of $154,400, just twice as much as pediatricians.

Insurers reimburse providers for medical services in various ways. The most common arrangement in the United States is "fee-for-service" (FFS), whereby a fee is charged for each separate service provided, such as a day in a hospital bed, a visit to a physician's office, or a specific laboratory test. Payment is made after services are received.

Paying the Hospital: Cost vs. Charge

In describing provider payment, "a distinction must be made between the *real-resource costs* of treating patients and the *monetary* transfers occasioned by the treatment. The real-resource costs of a treatment consist of time physicians and other health workers devote to it, and of supplies, equipment, brick and mortar used up in the process. The monetary costs are measured by the amount of money patients directly or indirectly funnel to the owners of these real resources. Clearly, these monetary costs can rise without a commensurate increase in real-resource costs. For example, if a cardiac surgeon decides to raise his or her fee for a coronary bypass from $5,000 to $8,000, only the monetary cost of the treatment rises; its real-resource cost does not" (Reinhardt 1985, p. 56C).

The difference between costs and charges is relevant because hospitals are reimbursed by some payers on a "cost-plus" basis. The *cost* refers to the direct cost of the specific service provided, as well as a percentage of the hospital's fixed or indirect costs such as labor, capital investment, and maintenance. Other indirect expenses, such as medical education and technology acquisition, have also been factored into some payers' cost formulas. The *plus* refers to the percentage the hospital will receive above and beyond its expenses.

From 1965 through 1983 the Medicare program paid hospitals on this basis, and Medicaid programs in many states continue to do so. The original Medicare Part A legislation stipulated that reimbursement was to cover service fees plus 2 percent: that is, hospitals were to receive a 2 percent mark-up on the costs they incurred. (A subsequent amendment removed the additional 2 percent.) This original arrangement was a result of a political compromise negotiated in 1965 between Congress and the hospital lobby. It reflects not only the political strength of the AHA and the AMA at the time, but the laissez-faire attitude of government and other third-party payers toward the health care industry.

In previous eras many insurers paid exactly what providers billed. Today this arrangement is much less common. Uninsured patients may be expected to pay their bills in full, although many are unable to; but third-party payers use a variety of seemingly arcane procedures to determine how much of the bill they will pay. Techniques differ, but all payers use the spread between costs and charges, between real-resource costs and monetary costs, as their basis for determining payments.

As in most markets, powerful buyers pay less per unit of product than less powerful buyers. As an insurer's market share (the number of persons it covers) increases, its ability to negotiate "discounted" payment levels also increases; by contrast, small in-surers and "self-pay" patients have no such bargaining leverage. This was not always as well understood as it is today. Thus al-though Medicare controlled a huge share of the market from its inception, policymakers did not effectively wield their potential power during the 1960s and exerted their influence only tenta-tively during the 1970s. But things have changed in this era of cost containment, as we shall see in the following chapter.

The same thing happens in the private sector. Whereas most commercial insurers must base their reimbursements largely on charges, the Blues, because of their market power nationally, can base theirs on costs. Also, because of the Blues' long-standing and close relationship with hospitals, many plans have reimburse-ment agreements with institutions that are highly dependent on Blues revenue. The resulting leverage strengthens the Blues' ability to offer competitive premiums.

Paying the Physician: UCR and CPR

Payers in an FFS system calculate reimbursement amounts in vari-ous ways. Three of the most common are the usual-customary-reasonable (UCR) method, the customary-prevailing-reasonable (CPR) method, and fee schedules. Whatever they are, or are not, most health care financing experts consider these existing pay-ment methods to be anything but "reasonable."

UCR and CPR are variations on a common theme. UCR was developed in the early 1960s by private insurance companies and later served as a model for developing the CPR formula, which is now used by Medicare Part B for the reimbursement of profes-sional fees and by many state Medicaid programs. Payers using these methods establish a multifactorial data base, known as the provider's payment history or profile, for all practitioners partici-pating in their program. As taken from this data base and other sources, these payment systems incorporate several components (Table 7).

In the private sector, most Blue Shield plans consider the 90th percentile of charges for a given service in a geographic area to be the prevailing (or customary) charge. Some insurance com-panies using UCR-CPR methodology use the 92nd percentile.

Table 7   **A Comparison of the Components of the UCR and CPR Physician Reimbursement Systems**

Component of methodology	"CPR" (used by Medicare)	"UCR" (used by private insurers)
Average past fee, based on individual physician's "historic fee profile"	Customary fee	Usual fee
Percentile (e.g., 75% or 90%) of the charges submitted by all physicians in a designated area for "similar" services	Prevailing fee	Customary fee
Charge submitted to insurer for service provided	Actual or submitted charge	Actual or submitted charge
Maximum allowable fee reimbursed to provider	Reasonable fee or approved charge ·	Reasonable fee or Reimbursed charge

Medicare Part B bases its prevailing fee on the 75th percentile, and limits are placed on yearly increases. These limits are determined on the basis of the Medicare Economic Index (MEI), a formula that considers a variety of economic factors including area-wide wage levels. Also, as of 1987 a second complex formula known as the Maximum Allowable Actual Charge (MAAC) is used by Medicare to cap the actual charges of "nonparticipating" providers.

Under Medicare's CPR method, in general, the "reasonable" or "approved" fee is the lesser of the customary, prevailing fee and the actual charge. After the patient's deductible has been met, Medicare pays 80 percent of this approved amount and the patient 20 percent. For private insurance companies under UCR, the reimbursed amount is the lesser of the usual, customary fee and the actual charge.

"Accepting assignment" is another feature of insurance reimbursement. A practitioner who chooses to accept assignment may submit bills directly to the insurer. Using the Medicare program as an example, such a practitioner agrees to accept the program's reimbursement amount as full payment for 80 percent of the service, with the patient responsible for the remaining 20 percent. If the physician does not accept assignment, the bill is sent to the patient, who is responsible not only for 20 percent coinsurance but for any amount that exceeds Medicare's approved fee. This practice is known as "balance-billing."

Currently physicians and other providers can become Medicare Participating Physicians by agreeing to accept assignment for all services and beneficiaries for one year. Alternatively they can decide to accept assignment on a case-by-case basis. Participating Physicians have been promised greater fee increases than nonparticipants in future years. For their part, patients obviously prefer to receive care from physicians who accept assignment, because this way their out-of-pocket costs are lower. In fiscal 1984 approximately 84 percent of nonfederal physicians accepted assignment for some percentage of their Medicare patients. In fiscal 1987 only 30 percent or so agreed to accept assignment for all Medicare patients. Since 1985 several states have passed laws *requiring* all physicians to accept assignment; other states will probably follow suit.

One serious drawback of the UCR-CPR payment method is that it encourages fee inflation. Not only do a practitioner's fees determine reimbursement in the present (as the "actual" component of the fee), but this year's fees determine next year's "customary" fees. Today's charge also influences an area's average prevailing fee level. When these "fee-padding" incentives are aggregated across all practitioners in an area, fees can become badly inflated. If patients complain, some providers explain that the fee on the bill is for the insurance company only; a second, lower, fee is what will actually be accepted for the patient's portion of the bill. (This arrangement is separate from the "sliding-fee schedule" that providers sometimes offer to low-income, uninsured patients.)

Another drawback of UCR-CPR reimbursement is that it offers no incentive to translate gains in efficiency into lower charges. For example, when a new lens extraction technique reduced the operating time for cataract surgery to an average of twenty minutes, ophthalmologists' fees generally remained at the "prevailing" levels set at a time when the procedure took much

longer and placed the patient at much higher risk. Reimbursement levels for this procedure and ten others were ultimately targeted by Medicare for downward adjustment.

Still another problem is that UCR-CPR is a complex process,
requiring, among other things, annual updating of the customary
and prevailing charges. Because fee levels are in continuous flux,
practitioners are rarely able to determine in advance how much
an insurer will pay for a given service. This is a disadvantage for
both patients and physicians.

Indeed, very different amounts might be paid at any one time
for the same service or a similar one, depending on the type of
practitioner or the delivery setting. "Under [Medicare's] CPR,
specialists tend to be remunerated at higher rates than generalists,
and urban-based practitioners at higher rates than those in rural
settings. Furthermore, reasonable payments for visits in hospital
settings and for consultations are usually greater than for office
visits" (Juba 1985a, p. 7).

If two or more practitioners provide the same services or services of similar complexity, should their reimbursement be the
same? A recent study found that even after adjustments were
made for complexity of the service, overhead, and other cost factors that could affect price, general practitioners were reimbursed
an average of $40 per hour as against $200 per hour for surgical
specialists. Most observers would probably agree that surgeons
deserve a higher hourly wage—but by a factor of five?

Table 8 shows some Medicare prevailing charges for specialists
and nonspecialists in 1982. For these services, specialists charged
from 24 to 73 percent more than nonspecialists. Similar price
differentials exist for most other services.

Fee Schedules

Problems with the UCR-CPR method have led to a renewed
interest in weighted fee schedules, whereby reimbursement is related to the complexity of the service provided and then set at a
fixed amount for all providing that service. Fee schedules eliminate some of the common pricing distortions found in the UCR-
CPR system.

Table 8   **Specialists' and Nonspecialists' Medicare Prevailing Charges for Five Common Services, 1982**

Service	Average charge		Difference (percent)
	Nonspecialist	Specialist	
Brief follow-up hospital visit	$16.63	$23.90	43.7%
Limited follow-up hospital visit	19.63	25.88	31.8
Limited follow-up office visit	16.99	21.05	23.9
Brief follow-up office visit	13.58	17.67	30.1
Minimal follow-up office visit	16.11	27.92	73.3

Source: U.S. Congress 1986, p. 108.

Some older fee schedules are not based on a specific valuation system, but are simply lists of amounts that will be paid as compensation under a health insurance policy, usually with minimal coverage. Many of these lists were developed on the basis of insurers' UCR experience. Other, more recent schedules are based on a more sophisticated approach to the relative weighting of different services. Usually termed RVU (for Relative Value Unit) or RVS (for Relative Value Scale) systems, these weighting schemes represent efforts to identify a homogeneous product within the heterogeneous care delivery process and to determine a fair value for that product.

A fundamental task in creating an RVS is identifying an appropriate dimension of worth and value. Variables used as bases for relative scales are physicians' charges, length of time spent providing care or doing a procedure, estimates of overhead costs and other costs of providing a service, and estimates of the degree of skill, the level of training, and the intensity of effort necessary to perform a service adequately. Developing an RVS is a complicated and value-laden process. Even something as seemingly straightforward as casting a leg is complex. Should a surgeon be paid on the basis of time spent? Skill? Degree of risk taken? Many nonsurgical encounters lead only to the exchange of information or the reassurance of the patient. How should results be measured? How reimbursed?

Once a weighting coefficient for each procedure or service is established, a dollar conversion factor is used to create a fee schedule; multiplying the weighting coefficient by the conversion factor yields a fee for that procedure. If necessary, additional elements such as geographic region, the physician's specialty, or the type of setting (hospital vs. office) can be factored in.

Despite their intricacy, many RVSs have been developed over the years, and fee schedules based on them have been used by Medicaid programs—25 in 1981—and by some commercial insurance companies. One of the best-known scales, the California Relative Value Scale (CRVS), has not been updated since 1974 as a result of a price-fixing suit brought against its developer, the California Medical Association. (Current antitrust law states that physician organizations cannot sponsor or derive RVSs.) But even before these legal difficulties surfaced, the CRVS system had been criticized for several inherent biases, notably putting excessive weight on the use of technology in patient care.

Despite drawbacks like these, RVSs have several advantages over the UCR-CPR method. Unlike UCR-CPR, the RVS approach has no built-in impetus for an automatic annual fee increase. If properly designed, an RVS will also minimize the price distortions intrinsic in the UCR-CPR method by permitting payers to retain some control over geographic variations in fee levels, the comparability of fees paid to generalists and specialists, and the relative value of technical and cognitive services.

HCFA-funded experts have been studying ways to develop an RVS system that would bring Medicare Part B pricing into conformity with national health policy goals, make payments more equitable, and direct providers' behavior toward efficency. Until such a system is devised and put into effect, we can only surmise what impact it would have on medical practice.

Capitation and Salary

Paying a physician by capitation or salary offers a major alternative to fee-for-service payment. In a capitation scheme a practitioner or a provider organization agrees to care for enrollees in return for an arranged per-capita fee. Historically these arrangements were first used by large group practices that became known as "prepaid group practices" (PPGPs). In areas where PPGPs gained a foothold, some solo physicians made their own prepayment arrangements as a way of maintaining an independent practice. These physicians often formed associations that were coordinated by local medical societies and were termed Independent (or Individual) Practice Associations (IPAs).

In 1972 the term "health maintenance organization" was applied by the Nixon Administration to both PPGPs and IPAs in the hope that this affirmative name would make capitation plans more palatable to skeptical patients and providers. Today many types of HMOs provide hospitalization, professional fees, and other covered services out of their revenue from prepaid premiums. Some HMO practitioners are paid by salary or receive a per capita payment; many others are paid on an FFS basis, and still others by a combination of FFS and capitation. Physicians on salary often receive a productivity-based incentive payment as well.

To encourage noncapitated practitioners to minimize their use of medical services, they almost always share some financial risk with the HMO. For example, some portion (say, 20 percent) of their FFS reimbursement may be "held back" until the end of the year, at which time it is determined whether their use of services during that year has been efficient. If inefficiencies are found—for example, excessive referral to specialists—part or all of the held-back amount may be kept by the HMO. Alternatively, the clinician may receive a percentage of the organization's profits at year's end.

Some contractual arrangements in HMOs are very complex and lead to correspondingly complex arrangements for reimbursement. For example, a physician may be a member of a small private group practice that subcontracts to a larger group, which in turn contracts to several distinct HMOs, each using a somewhat different payment scheme. In fact, there are almost as many ways to arrange reimbursement within an HMO as there are HMOs.

Many salaried physicians are employed by institutions other than HMOs, among them hospitals and health centers. *Recent surveys indicate that over half of U.S. physicians receive at least some of their income as a basic salary.* This statistic reflects not only the growth of HMOs but also an increase in non-HMO group practice arrangements, which often place younger partners on full or partial salary. (Some implications of this trend are discussed in Part II.)

Providers' Incentives and Reimbursement Methods

It has been estimated that physicians make direct decisions affecting 70 to 90 percent of all health care outlays. Thus, although they receive only about 20 percent of such outlays themselves, their practices have an immense influence over the rest. Different payment mechanisms offer practitioners different incentives, and these incentives may significantly influence the amount and type of care a patient receives.

FFS reimbursement, the predominant method, invites the provider to offer as many services as the patient's condition could possibly warrant. FFS rewards providers for keeping patients in the hospital, perhaps longer than necessary, and ensuring that they receive every conceivable test and treatment up to the levels of available technology and insurance coverage. *The simplicity of the FFS concept belies its power to inflate costs. Some economists argue that this is the major cause of increasing health care expenditures.*

Similarly, cost-plus reimbursement contains no strong financial incentive for hospitals to be managed efficiently, since any increase in a hospital's operating cost is passed along to payers in the form of higher charges. Even when effective management, increased patient volume, technological improvements, or increased provider skills reduce costs, charges are rarely lowered.

The capitation arrangement offers a different constellation of economic incentives. First, the provider organization and its individual practitioners bear the financial risk instead of the third-party payer or consumer. Second, because the capitation payment depends only on the number of people cared for, rather than on the quantity of services, there is no incentive to maximize the volume of services provided. Indeed, there is some incentive to enroll more members and do less for each.

Salaried practitioners, like those in capitation plans, receive no financial reward for increasing the number of services provided; but unlike those in capitation plans they are also not usually rewarded financially for caring for an increased number of patients. For these reasons some economists regard the salary method as the most neutral type of reimbursement.

Cost savings in capitation and salary systems seem to come largely from lower physician-induced demand. In fact, because capitation offers physicians an incentive to provide less care, there has been considerable concern that HMO patients would not be well served. Extensive research in the 1960s and 1970s, however, showed that by and large HMO patients receive care equal or superior to that received by FFS patients. The differences were not so much qualitative as quantitative: enrollees in prepaid HMOs received more ambulatory care and less surgery than FFS patients and were hospitalized less often.

As part of the Rand Health Insurance Experiment, groups of people were randomly assigned to an HMO and several FFS plans; the random assignment process eliminated any possibility that HMO cost advantages, if found, might be attributable to a self-selection of healthier people into HMOs. The FFS groups' health care expenditures were found to be more costly, largely because the HMO group's hospitalization rate was 40 percent lower. Since other potentially intervening variables were strictly controlled, the difference in costs between the two systems appears to be attributable largely to differences in physicians' incentives to hospitalize patients.

Another study in New England compared ten FFS physicians with seventeen HMO physicians with respect to ordering ECGs and chest x-rays, which are both high-cost and high-profit tests. It was found that on average the FFS practitioners ordered 50 percent more ECGs and 40 percent more chest x-rays than the HMO practitioners.

Alternative reimbursement methods have also been shown to affect surgeons' inclination to operate in borderline situations, with FFS reimbursement leading to higher rates of surgery. One study found surgery rates in capitation plans to be 3.5 to 5 per thousand, compared with 6.5 to 7 per thousand in FFS arrangements. A study of federal employees found that surgical procedures in capitation plans were performed at one-fourth to one-half the rate of the same procedures in FFS plans.

Physicians in the United Kingdom are part of a national health service under which GPs are paid primarily by capitation and specialists by salary. Comparative studies have found, among other things, that United Kingdom physicians perform surgery at about one-half the rate of United States physicians, and perform fewer radiological studies. Such comparisons, to be meaningful, must be correlated with comparative data on the health status of the two populations and the quality and outcome of care; otherwise it cannot be said for sure whether Americans pay too much for health care or pay what may be a reasonable price for higher-quality care. Arguments both ways have nonetheless been made for decades.

Today, however, with numerous studies showing unnecessary inefficiencies throughout the health care delivery system, payers and policymakers seem to have reached a consensus that changes are necessary in the reimbursement of providers. Recently the Medicare program has led the way in developing innovative reimbursement methods. The following chapter describes what has been and is being done to make providers' behavior more cost-effective.

CHAPTER 7

COSTS: THE PAYER'S PERSPECTIVE

The role of third-party payers has so increased in recent years that such payers are thought by many to exert more influence on health care practice than either patients or providers. Understanding payers' objectives, which include maximizing revenue and minimizing expenditures, is therefore critical to understanding today's health care delivery process.

Actions taken by payers to influence the behavior of hospital administrators and physicians fall into two overlapping categories: regulatory and competitive. Regulatory interventions seek to prescribe or prohibit certain kinds of behavior by providers. Competitive interventions neither prescribe nor prohibit, but instead offer incentives designed to encourage cost-sensitive competitive behavior.

Planning: A Regulatory Approach

Most developed countries have central agencies at the national or regional level that control medical care resources and coordinate their allocation. By contrast, the pluralistic United States has decentralized planning agencies, and these agencies have been at best only modestly successful in influencing investment in health care. Profitability considerations have generally been paramount in determining such investment. As a result, some areas today are burdened with surplus facilities while others (usually rural or inner-city areas) remain underequipped.

In the 1960s, after the introduction of Medicare and Medicaid, the federal government sought ways of containing costs by preventing unnecessary capital expansion. Despite the opposition of powerful political groups such as the AMA and the AHA, sporadic efforts at regional planning were made; and in the mid-1970s the Federal Planning Act authorized the creation of a large-scale network of local and regional agencies to plan for the health care needs of communities and states. These consumer-dominated semigovernmental units, which came to be known as Health Systems Agencies (HSAs) and State Health Planning and Development Agencies, had considerable say in the certification process for major capital expansion within existing health care facilities, but had no authority to halt non-capital-intensive projects that their planners deemed unnecessary. Moreover, providers could ignore the agencies' suggestions regarding what new programs were needed by the community. As a result, they had only modest impact on the growth of the health care sector in most areas before they fell victim to the Reagan Administration's budget cuts in 1986.

The so-called Certificate-of-Need (CON) program, mandated by Congress as part of the Planning Act and still in effect in most states, is controlled by state planning units with assistance from local HSAs where present. The program requires hospitals and other medical institutions to obtain a "certificate of need" from the state before purchasing major equipment, developing new services, or making other capital investments beyond a certain minimum. Over time this minimum has increased from about $100,000 to $1 million or more in many states. Planning boards determine whether proposed investments are necessary and have the authority to turn down projects deemed unnecessary. Although the Reagan Administration relaxed the rules for this program, in 1987 some 42 states still had either a CON process, an equivalent program, or a moratorium on new hospital construction and expansion projects.

A number of difficulties arose with the CON process. Many hospitals found innovative ways to skirt the regulations. Moreover, because planning boards invariably included physicians and hospital administrators as well as local citizens (the majority), all of whom benefited from an investment in state-of-the-art medicine, these bodies only rarely opposed new construction projects. For all these reasons, the Planning Act did little to control investment in health care facilities.

Utilization Control: A Regulatory Approach

In contrast to planning, which is used to control capital investments, utilization control seeks to achieve efficiency in the basic unit of service, the patient-practitioner encounter. In utilization review (UR), physicians' actual use of health care resources is examined case by case in the light of predetermined criteria. When these criteria are set by the same physicians being monitored, the review is usually termed a "peer review," even if the actual reviewer is a nurse or a medical records technician. To date, UR programs have concentrated on limiting the "unnecessary" use of health care resources rather than on improving the outcome of care. Although a reasonably solid argument can be made that limiting unneeded care will have a positive effect on the patient's outcome of care, at some point further reductions will clearly have the opposite effect.

The decisions most often scrutinized in UR programs are whether to hospitalize a patient, how long to keep a patient in the hospital, and whether to perform a major therapeutic procedure such as surgery or a major diagnostic procedure such as angiography or CT scan. A review can take place before the event (prospective), at the time of the event (concurrent), or after the event (retrospective).

By stiffening criteria and disallowing reimbursements when established standards are not met, UR becomes a cost control measure. To the extent that it induces errant physicians to mend their ways, it can also be used as a quality assurance mechanism.

UR was first developed in the 1930s as part of an effort to improve the quality of care. It became prominent as a cost control tool only after the enactment of Medicare and Medicaid, when federal law mandated a review of hospital and physician reimbursement "to avert overservicing in the Medicare and Medicaid programs—e.g. unjustified surgery, which might be both harmful and costly" (Roemer 1982, p. 33). Hospitals were at first put in charge of their own reviews, but this self-regulation was found to be ineffective and gave way in 1972 to review by Professional Standards Review Organizations (PSROs).

PSROs, composed of local physicians, were founded in 187

geographic areas and were supported by the federal government to review hospital admissions and length of stay for beneficiaries of the Medicare, Medicaid, and Maternal and Child Health programs. They were to identify unnecessary admissions and hospital days, for which reimbursement would be denied, and could also recommend sanctions against individual physicians. As the first major program to monitor the actual delivery of care, the PSRO system was a harbinger of future trends.

The PSRO legislation was promoted to physicians as a way of improving the quality of care, and to Congress as a means of cost control. The two purposes may in fact be consistent (this hotly debated issue is discussed further in Part II), but in this case their potential divergence created confusion from the start. The program was also plagued by administrative difficulties, was inadequately supported by practitioners, and showed no clear signs of effectiveness. For these reasons and others the PSROs were terminated in 1982 and replaced by similar entities known as Peer Review Organizations (PROs).

In the PRO system, one independent group in each state—often a reborn PSRO—was awarded a contract to do the review work. To qualify, they were required to show either sponsorship or support by physicians, and they could not be associated with a health care facility or a third-party payer. PROs review only Medicare beneficiaries; Medicaid reviews are no long supported by the federal program, although some PROs do have separate state contracts for this purpose.

Like their predecessors, PROs were given a mix of cost and quality goals. Some of their major objectives were to encourage a shift of care from inpatient to outpatient settings, to decrease the number of invasive procedures and of complications from such procedures, to cut down on readmissions, and to improve the accuracy of diagnostic reporting and coding on medical records. Because programs varied widely both in their choice of what to monitor and in their goals or targets, such matters are now to a large extent federally mandated.

Although the PRO program is considered by many to be an improvement over its predecessor, difficulties remain: notably, the possibility that inaccurate data will lead to inaccurate conclusions, the concern that reputations may suffer unjustly from the 20/20 hindsight fostered by retrospective review, and the lack of an adequate mechanism to deal with disagreements between reviewers and practitioners regarding the management of a case. Despite these drawbacks, PRO programs seem likely to serve as the principal public-sector utilization review and quality assurance method for the near future.

When private health insurance companies began operating in the 1930s, they did not monitor the use of resources by hospitals or physicians. This changed with the advent of Medicare, when many private insurers became "fiscal intermediaries" for the program. Not only did they provide administrative services, such as handling claim forms and making payments to beneficiaries and providers, but more generally they acted as conduits between government, consumers, and providers. They were also responsible for monitoring claims and payments and acting on the findings of the PSROs.

Many insurance companies adopted the Medicare review methods for their own policyholders. This surveillance has increased over the years to the point where many companies are now involved in aggressive UR activities, questioning physicians' decisions and even specifying norms of practice. Some term this the "managed-care" phenomenon, involving as it does the managing of physicians' behavior as well as of health care resources.

Today there are a range of UR approaches. One is preadmission certification, in which a review organization acting as proxy for the insurer grants permission for a patient to be hospitalized, failing which payment will be denied. Another is concurrent review, in which the review organization monitors a hospital patient's progress to determine if continued inpatient care is medically necessary.

A similar approach, although not technically a review program, is to pay for certain surgical procedures only if they are performed on an outpatient basis (known as "same day" or ambulatory surgery). As we have seen, the Medicare program has an extensive list of such procedures, which include small skin grafts, rectal polypectomy, tubal ligation, and gynecologic laparoscopy. Payment can even be denied after the service has been performed and billed, for example if a physician hospitalizes a patient to perform a skin graft and cannot prove that unusual circumstances required inpatient treatment. The patient is also usually exempt from responsibility for payment in such cases.

Businesses now are also using UR programs to control health benefit costs. The number of corporations mandating preadmission review for employees increased from 2 percent in 1982 to 26 percent in 1984. Many employers now require their insurance carriers to set up such programs; others operate UR programs themselves or contract with independent reviewer or "managed care" organizations (see next chapter). This has become a booming business for many defunded PSROs.

Regulatory Approaches to Reimbursement

Since it is now clear that reimbursement methods can influence clinical decisions, modifying the reimbursement process is another way used by third parties to affect medical decision-making. Resolute policymakers now consider payment mechanisms central to the problem of inducing providers to improve their decision-making. The general premise is that if providers can be made more cognizant of the resources they control, they will assume some responsibility for the costs they generate.

Rate-setting of one sort or another has been tried several times by government during the cost containment era. Unlike certificate-of-need and other regulations designed to control providers' investments, rate-setting controls the prices they may charge. Price freezes and payment caps have been the principal strategies of this type.

From 1971 to 1974 the Nixon Administration attempted to control rampant economy-wide inflation with the Economic Stabilization Act, which included a 90-day wage and price freeze on all providers. This worked reasonably well during the program's existence: per-day and per-admission hospital costs decreased, and the annual rate of increase of physicians' fees fell from 7.4 percent to 2.4 percent. But when the program was discontinued, price inflation resumed at its previous steep rate.

In 1972, as we have seen, Congress limited increases in physicians' fees for Medicare patients by subjecting them to the Medicare Economic Index. Under this complex formula, yearly increases are based on increases in the cost of practice and in general wage levels. In some years Congress has voted to allow no increase at all. A fifteen-month freeze declared in 1984 was extended several times: ultimately to May 1, 1986, for Participating Physicians and December 31, 1986, for nonparticipating physicians. Starting in 1987, the prevailing-charge increases of nonparticipating physicians lagged one year behind those of Participating Physicians.

Practitioners responded to these fee freezes by various kinds of "game-playing," notably reclassifying services into higher-paying categories, "unbundling" a single-charge service into separate billable units, and providing more units of service. It has been argued that physicians have a so-called "target income" and simply modify their behavior as necessary to assure that this income is reached. However this may be, economists generally agree that freezes and caps have not been effective cost control measures.

Capitation

As noted earlier, President Nixon's advisers were convinced of the cost-saving potential of capitation plans and supported the development of such plans. The HMO Act, passed in 1973, specified federal qualifications for HMOs, among them a minimum benefit package, a quality-of-care review process, and regulations to ensure sound financial backing. Employers with more than 25 employees were required to offer an HMO option if there was a federally qualified plan in their area. This legislation was intended to encourage competition among HMO plans, and between HMOs and traditional insurance plans.

HMO regulations were made strict in response to the fear that HMOs might provide inferior medical care because of their financing structure. They were also required to offer far more comprehensive benefits than most traditional insurance policies of the time. This increased costs, and the resulting higher premiums probably hindered the growth of HMO plans. Although businesses began offering such plans to their employees, the high premiums dissuaded many from signing up and there was no dramatic increase in the aggregate enrollment in capitated plans.

Price Discounting

In this era of cost control, third-party payers are becoming "prudent buyers," demanding discounts or looking for new providers who are willing to accept lower fees.

Discounts can be arranged in many ways. Payer and provider may negotiate a contract stipulating discounted fees; the Blues have traditionally negotiated such contracts with hospitals. Providers may submit competitive bids to serve a given patient population; payers accepting the lowest bid have in effect been offered a price discount. Some employers have purchased plans for their employees that incorporate discounts negotiated by insurance companies; others have negotiated their own discounts. The California Medicaid program (Medi-Cal) recently reduced its expenditures by requiring hospitals and other providers to submit closed bids for contracts to provide care for the state's medical assistance patients.

A surplus of physicians and hospital beds has created a buyer's market for health care. The resulting contracts benefit not only payers but providers, who, in return for their discount, are guaranteed a certain volume of patients at a time when many hospitals and physicians are competing for the consumer's dollar. As part of a discount deal, many payers also agree to expedite payment, which otherwise is rarely swift.

Discounting is the basis of new arrangements known as preferred provider organizations (PPOs). In a PPO, employers or insurers offer their beneficiaries significant incentives to use certain preferred sources of care and these providers in turn offer discounts (often 20 percent) from their conventional fees. The PPO entity agrees to accept a degree of accountability by establishing a strong UR program. Because providers under PPO arrangements receive fee-for-service payment, they do not bear the financial risk that is associated with an HMO arrangement.

Patients enrolled in PPOs are usually not *required* to obtain care from the preferred group, but are rewarded for doing so. In general, the incentives for enrollees involve extra services (such as preventive care) or waived co-payments and deductibles; enrollees remain free to consult other providers who do not offer such incentives. In a variant of the PPO, known as the exclusive provider organization, the patient may not readily seek care outside the PPO system. (There is more on PPOs in the next chapter.)

The Medicare Prospective Payment System

In 1983, the financing of Medicare Part A was radically restructured when Congress introduced the Prospective Payment System (PPS). Under PPS, a hospital is paid a prospectively determined, fixed amount per patient admission regardless of how many services the patient receives. *This legislation represents the most significant departure in the financing (and consequently in the delivery) of U.S. health care since the inception of the Medicare program itself.*

PPS applies to hospital inpatient services only, which were chosen as a starting point because they are the single most expensive component (over 50 percent) of aggregate federal spending on health care. The purpose of PPS was to keep Medicare costs down by setting the annual spending level for U.S. acute-care hospitals in advance. Under PPS each patient admission is assigned to a category via a system known as Diagnosis Related Groups (DRGs); hence PPS is often termed the DRG System.

DRGs are based on the International Classification of Diseases, 9th revision (ICD-9) coding system, a taxonomy of about 10,000 diagnoses and 5,000 procedure codes. In the early 1970s Yale University researchers classified hospital patients into groups on the basis of diagnoses, procedures, and age as a way of explaining variations in their resource use and length of stay in the hospital. The outcome was approximately 390 DRGs. This classification was revised in 1979, and now includes 468 categories. Figure 11 graphically depicts how patients with primary conditions related to blood and blood formation are grouped into one of eight DRGs based on their diagnoses, procedures, and age.

Under PPS each DRG is assigned a coefficient representing the resource intensity deemed necessary to care for a patient assigned to that DRG. This coefficient is multiplied by a dollar amount to convert it to a price, and this is the fee paid to the hospital for a given patient in that DRG. If the hospital's costs for that patient

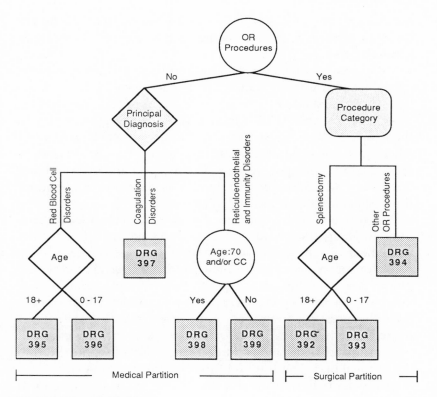

Fig. 11. A major diagnostic category (MDC) of the Diagnosis Related Group (DRG) case-mix system: Diseases and disorders of the blood and blood-forming organs and immunological disorders. (Source: HCFA 1983.)

exceed the fee, the hospital will lose money on the patient; if the fee exceeds its costs, it will make a profit. Since a particular hospital is paid on the basis of its entire mix of cases, the DRG payment scheme is sometimes known as a "case-mix" or per-case reimbursement system.

PPS was originally designated as a "budget-neutral" reimbursement method because in its first year it was not intended to reduce expenditures. Such a system does make tight control possible, however, since if spending in year x exceeds accepted levels the dollar multiplier can be decreased for year $x + 1$. This downward ratcheting mechanism has already been applied by Medicare administrators.

Prospective payment rates for a given DRG are determined by several factors, among them the cost of a typical Medicare inpatient day (based on accounting audits) and relative resource requirements for that DRG (figured in terms of length of stay in the hospital). Reimbursement for "outlier patients," so named when their hospital bill reaches 150 percent of, or $12,000 more than, the DRG prospective price, has also been incorporated into the system. Medicare pays 60 percent of the hospital bill above the outlier cutoff amount.

PPS was phased in gradually. In its initial stages local variations in charges were incorporated into payments as a further refinement of separate urban and rural rates. Adjustments were made for sole community hospitals, regional referral centers, and cancer hospitals. But these adjustments were gradually phased out, and by 1988 hospitals were paid national rates, adjusted only for differences in average area wage levels, teaching status, and degree to which they *disproportionately* care for the indigent. Chronic, psychiatric, and children's hospitals were excluded from the original plan, and this exclusion has remained in effect.

One potential problem with the PPS system is that it rewards providers financially for maximizing hospital admissions. Yet in fact Medicare admissions have *decreased* since PPS, continuing a trend that began before PPS was introduced. Some analysts think that the continuing decline may be partly due to the influence of Peer Review Organizations, since every PPS admission comes under PRO review.

When PPS was introduced in 1983, several states were exempted because they already had similar reimbursement systems in place for all payers. Maryland, New Jersey, New York, and Massachusetts, all with very high hospital charges and length-of-stay figures compared to national averages, instituted such "all-payer" rate controls early. As a result, they have held rises in health care costs several points below the national average. For example, whereas in 1977 Maryland's hospital costs were 20 percent higher than the national average, by 1985 they were only 1 percent higher. In that year Maryland recorded greater decreases in hospital admissions and length of hospital stay than the United States as a whole.

States may remain exempt from PPS as long as average Medicare payments in the state do not surpass the national average. New Jersey will remain exempt at least through 1988. New York and Massachusetts decided to drop their exemption rather than try to meet the standard. In 1988 Maryland policymakers hoped to remain in exempt status because they believe that their system leads to more efficient treatment not just of Medicare patients but of all patients.

Several state Medicaid programs have introduced PPS, and by 1985 as many as 33 states had some degree of PPS for medical assistance patients. Some are using DRGs to group discharge diagnoses; others rely on alternative methods. Although some Blues plans also use PPS (with and without DRGs), as of 1988 the great majority of privately insured hospital patients were not admitted under a PPS plan.

As discounting and prospective payment become important aspects of health care financing, "cost-shifting" between different types of payers increases in significance as a policy issue. An estimated 13 percent of a private patient's bill now pays costs shifted from the bills of patients covered by public programs or discount arrangements. For example, because PPS limits the percent of overhead it will cover, nonregulated payers have been charged higher prices. Such practices anger private insurers; they prefer all-payer systems (such as in Maryland), which make it impossible to shift costs to the private sector. The profound effects of PPS on hospitals and physicians, as well as other problems with the system, are explored in later chapters.

Future Expansion of Prospective Payment to Other Providers

DRG-based prospective payment currently applies only to the facility's portion of a hospital charge. It does not extend to Medicare Part B, the professional service component of the program, which currently accounts for about one-third of all Medicare expenditures and will soon become the third-largest federal social program, behind Social Security and Medicare Part A. About 75 percent of Part B payments are for physicians' services. As of 1984, Part B expenditures were increasing at an annual rate of 16 percent, over four times as fast as the overall inflation rate (see Table 4, p. 57). In an effort to bring this alarming increase under control, policymakers are now exploring ways of applying some type of DRG-like method to physicians' reimbursement under Medicare Part B.

Just as hospital services have been bundled for payment purposes, there has been a trend toward looking at the patient "as a package." In capitation systems, for example, a year's worth of patient care is bundled into one prepaid fee. There appears to be no inherent obstacle to PPS bundling of physicians' services for both inpatient and ambulatory care, or of nursing home care.

Surgeons and obstetricians are already paid for some of their services by the bundle; for example, pre- and post-operative visits are usually included in the surgical fee. Other specialists do not bundle their services, and equitable payment methods for them are still undetermined. Some experts have called for a per-case approach, known as MD-DRGs, whereby an admitting physician would received a flat fee to provide all hospital-based care.

A variation on this MD-DRG bundling approach would move beyond the admitting physician to encompass all physician services provided during an admission, including radiology, anesthesia, and pathology (the so-called "RAP" services), surgery, and consultations, as well as hospital visits by the attending physician. This package fee could be paid either to the hospital, which would negotiate a payment arrangement with physicians, to the medical staff, which would apportion it, or to the attending physician, who would pay the specialists used in the case. Another issue is whether fees should cover the spectrum from outpatient to inpatient to long-term care, thereby preventing practitioners from shifting treatment locations to collect extra fees. Arguments for and against all these arrangements have been made. A researcher comments as follows: "Packaging physician services restores much of the burden to the physician making the decision, as with any entrepreneur. Under a physician DRG system, the decision to bring in a consultant carries with it specific cost consequences for the physician since these additional costs must come out of a fixed case payment" (Mitchell 1985b, p. 10).

When the discharge records of hospitalized Medicare patients in four states were used to test the MD-DRG concept by grouping patients into potential categories, those within *medical* MD-DRGs had a far higher variation in their present physician charges than those in *surgical* MD-DRGs. This suggests that it may be more difficult to develop a fair per-case reimbursement system for nonsurgical specialties.

Furthermore, in this study the average physician admitted only 2–2.5 Medicare patients per DRG, and treated patients in 15–18 different DRGs per year. Since the DRG system works on the principle that a large number of patients within a given category cancels the effects of a few outliers, many believe that the small numbers found in this exploratory study rule out the compensation of individual physicians on a DRG basis. Predictably, it is argued, some physicians would enjoy windfall profits under such a system, and others would experience relative hardship. Because larger numbers would in theory solve this problem, some analysts feel that multispecialty group practices may be ideal for experimenting with per-case DRG-like payment arrangements. There are over 3,500 multispecialty group practices in the United States, averaging more than nine physicians per group. Many such practices, it is argued, have large enough patient populations to spread the risk adequately.

Another important drawback to MD-DRGs from the providers' perspective is that any such system would probably require them to accept mandatory assignment, which would mean accepting the Medicare fee as payment in full for all patients.

Because of all these complicating factors HCFA has decided against using MD-DRG reimbursement on a national basis, at least for now, appearing instead to favor a fee-schedule approach based on a revised relative value scale. Among other things, physicians seem likely to prefer such an arrangement to MD-DRG reimbursement.

In addition to PPS approaches for physician services in the hospital setting, other PPS schemes are in planning stages or have been introduced on a limited basis. One such scheme is a case-mix approach for ambulatory visits designed by the developers of DRGs and known as Ambulatory Visit Groups (AVGs). This system, which has not yet been applied by any major payer, is based on ICD-9 diagnosis codes and on the Current Procedural Terminology (CPT) codes developed by the AMA. Because the AVG approach has problems similar to those of MD-DRGs, it is uncertain whether AVGs will be adopted by Medicare.

As the percentage of elderly persons in the population increases, so does the importance to both payers and providers of finding effective ways to control the costs of long-term care. A reimbursement method for nursing home care known as Resource Utilization Groups (RUGs) has been introduced in New York and elsewhere; like the DRGs this system pays the facility a preset fee based on the patient case-mix. It is likely that RUGs, or something similar to them, will gain favor with both the Medicare and Medicaid programs, which together pay about half of all nursing home costs.

Regardless of specifics, present trends indicate that FFS will in due course give way to one or another far-reaching reimbursement system featuring new incentives. The following chapter explores the impact of these and other cost control measures on the new medical marketplace.

CHAPTER 8

THE CHANGING MEDICAL MARKETPLACE

The 1983 Medicare DRG-based prospective payment legislation fueled competitive pressures that had been simmering in the health care industry pressure-cooker since the 1970s. This chapter explores some of these factors and describes the new competitive milieu in which today's providers practice.

It has been said that the health care industry was motivated in the 1960s by the "access imperative," grew in the 1970s because of the "technological imperative," and was driven in the 1980s by the "managerial imperative" (Iglehart 1985). Financial survival has required significant changes in the organization, management, and ownership of health care facilities, in relationships between the various participants in health care, and in health care itself. A transformation is under way, rivaling the transformation that followed the publication of the Flexner Report in 1910 and the introduction of Medicare and Medicaid in 1966.

The New Role of the Hospital

Hospital admissions began to decline in 1982, and the decline soon accelerated. *Aggregate U.S. hospital admissions decreased 4.8 percent from 1984 to 1985; there were 7.5 percent fewer inpatient days, and average length of stay in the hospital decreased 2.8 percent. The occupancy rate of community hospital beds fell from 74 percent in early 1983 to only 63 percent in mid-1985.* Clearly hospitals must now compete for a shrinking patient market, which is why we now see hospital advertising on television and billboards.

As expected, Congress has used PPS to control Medicare's hospital reimbursements. In both 1983 and 1984 the payment rate was increased by 4.15 percent annually; but in 1985 it was increased only 0.5 percent, even though HCFA estimated that hospitals' costs had risen by more than 11 percent during that year.

Many analysts predicted that PPS reimbursement would cause hospitals severe financial losses. That has not happened across the board, *but some 18,000 hospital beds were closed in 1985 and an estimated 18 percent of all hospitals are operating in the red.* Perhaps half of this 18 percent will close over the next few years, with small urban and rural hospitals the most likely to do so. There has also been a steady decrease in full-time-equivalent hospital employees beginning in 1983.

On the other hand, in 1985 many hospitals earned record profits under PPS reimbursement. Profits for the hospital industry as a whole rose to $2.8 billion in the first quarter of that year, a 22 percent increase over the first quarter of 1984 and the steepest percentage increase since the 1960s. A recent government survey of 900 hospitals showed an annual profit margin of approximately 14 percent even though 18 percent of the hospitals incurred losses. The AHA has reported a more modest average profit margin of approximately 6 percent for the industry, but both sources agree that profit margins have increased significantly.

For-Profit Medicine

Attention to the bottom line is not new to the American health care system; what *is* new is that today many hospitals' very survival may be at stake. Unlike the directors of the charity-run facilities of the early 1900s, today's hospital manager must have a high degree of business acumen.

Most hospitals are owned by nonprofit, tax-exempt entities whose surplus revenue is reinvested back into the organization rather than paid out as dividends to owners or investors. Yet it is clear from the profit margins reported above that a well-run hospital is a potentially profitable investment. As entrepreneurs and Wall Street investors have come to recognize this, investment in for-profit, investor-owned health care facilities has grown. Although such facilities have not significantly increased as a percentage of the industry since the 1960s, *between 1976 and 1984 the number of acute-care medical/surgical beds owned by for-profit corporations more than doubled, from 55,000 to 111,000.*

Some for-profit facilities are owner-operated; others are part of investor-owned multifacility systems. The concerns of most critics of for-profit medicine focus on the latter: "Because of their size, resources (both economic and political), ambitious growth strategies, and centralized control of multiple institutions, the importance of the investor-owned hospital companies should not be minimized; they are to the old 'doctor's hospitals' what agribusiness is to the family farm" (Gray 1986, p. 1525).

Arnold Relman has coined the label "medical-industrial complex" to describe the for-profit sector of the health care industry. Today for-profit, investor-owned corporations operate approximately 1,000 hospitals, 300 HMOs, 1,500 independent "convenience care" clinics, more than 11,000 nursing homes (approximately 77 percent of the total), and many other health care facilities. In 1987 more than 15 percent of nongovernmental acute-care hospitals and 50 percent of psychiatric hospitals were proprietary. In addition, numerous home care agencies, diagnostic laboratories, hemodialysis centers, mobile CT scanners, and other types of delivery organizations are part of the for-profit sector. In total such organizations receive approximately 15–20 percent of all health care expenditures, and the largest ones have annual sales in the billions of dollars. It is estimated that the five largest control over two-thirds of all investor-owned hospitals. (Some concerns that have been raised about the growth of for-profit medicine are discussed in Part II.)

Integration of Providers

Another recent trend is toward consolidation. Health care facilities too inefficient or inflexible to survive in the new environment are being acquired by or merged with more successful facilities to form multifacility systems. This process, termed *horizontal integration*, is occurring in both the for-profit and nonprofit sectors. The resulting arrangement is analogous to a chain of restaurants: one organization owns a number of facilities that provide the same type of service. In 1988 over one-third of all community hospitals were part of multihospital systems.

Because of pressure from payers to minimize inpatient care, hospital administrators expect to be asked to provide a narrower range of services in the future. To offset the concomitant loss of income, many hospitals are already offering prehospital care (such as ambulatory services) and posthospital care (such as long-term care). As part of this attempt to provide "cradle to grave" services, hospitals are purchasing or merging with nursing homes, psychiatric hospitals, outpatient surgery centers, and other facilities, and are setting up satellite outpatient centers and HMO networks. This type of expansion is known as *vertical integration*: one legal entity operates a group of facilities that together offer a broad range of services. In essence, the hospital is once again becoming the place for treating acute and severe diseases or for major surgery, with other services deemphasized or moved to off-site locations.

In a further integration of subsectors of the health care system, hospitals are selling health insurance policies. For example, the Humana Corporation, a large owner of hospitals, has sold group policies to thousands of corporate employers and now insures hundreds of thousands of workers. And conversely many insurance companies are becoming health care providers by acquiring or forming their own HMOs and PPOs, or by investing in or operating hospital chains. In short, medical providers and insurers—of which many, if not most, are for-profit corporations—are increasingly offering the same services and thus competing with each other.

Analysts believe that soon a handful of such integrated companies—termed "Super-Meds" by Paul Ellwood, who also coined the term "Health Maintenance Organization"—may control a majority of U.S. health care delivery. In the extreme outcome: "If current trends continue, the number of major parties involved in the health care enterprise will be reduced to only two. The new first party will be the governmental or business purchaser of health care, and the new second party will be the nationwide suppliers of health care—the megacorporate health care delivery systems" (Freedman 1985, p. 580).

Alternative Delivery Systems

The two main alternative delivery systems (also termed by some "managed-care" systems) are HMOs and PPOs. In 1988 there were over 700 HMOs in the country, with over 29 million members. These plans are growing at a rapid rate—over 250 percent since 1983—and have become increasingly popular with employers as well as with Medicare and Medicaid officials.

Although no two HMOs are quite alike, there are four broad types of HMOs. There is the Staff Model, in which physicians are directly employed by the organization on a salaried basis. There is the Group Model, in which a large group practice, corporately separate from the HMO, contractually provides the care. There is the Independent Practice Association (IPA) Model, in which solo practitioners or small groups agree to see HMO patients in addition to their FFS patients. And there is the Network Model, in which an HMO contracts with two or more larger groups to provide care to their patients.

In addition, HCFA has funded several experiments with an interesting new type of HMO, dubbed the Social HMO (or S/HMO), which is designed to serve the elderly by integrating the services of the typical HMO with long-term care, notably home care and nursing home care. Today most HMO plans, like indemnity plans, do not cover long-term care; but as the U.S. population ages and long-term care costs become an ever larger proportion of health care expenditures, there will be increasing pressure to find ways of paying those costs on a capitation basis.

The rapid growth of HMOs is thought likely to decrease the nation's need for new physicians, at least in the short term, because HMOs and other types of organized medical care delivery seemingly provide equal-quality care with fewer physicians than under FFS arrangements. Recent projections indicate that even fewer new physicians may be necessary over the next decade or so than experts had previously estimated.

A close cousin of the HMO, the preferred provider organization (PPO), is also undergoing explosive growth. As of 1988 over 570 plans were offering care to more than 35 million consumers—both figures up by several hundred percent since 1983. PPOs may be operated by insurance companies, independent entrepreneurs, hospitals, or physician groups—or by some combination of these sponsors, as in the Medical Staff and Hospital (MeSH) PPO, where a hospital and a collection of physicians jointly form a corporate entity. "Meshing," it is claimed, gives both groups incentives to work in tandem to achieve an efficent delivery process.

PPOs have been able to expand rapidly by capitalizing on providers' desires to retain market share and payers' desires to reduce costs, but the future of such organizations is not yet clear. Critics not only question whether discounting can go on forever, but fear that in the absence of prepayment or risk-sharing incentives practitioners will continue to provide more services than necessary. Some believe that PPOs will take over some of the prepayment market or possibly introduce some risk-sharing provisions, thereby blurring the line between PPOs and IPA-model HMOs. *Several well-known analysts believe that by 1990 half of all Americans may be HMO or PPO members. If PPOs and HMOs do succeed to that extent, they will affect medical practice dramatically. Among other things, all physicians will be either in one of the so-called "three-letter" health plans or competing with one; and in either case an efficient practice style will be essential.*

As a means of retaining their market share against HMOs and PPOs by improving their own cost efficiency, private indemnity insurance companies have taken to offering "managed indemnity plans" (MIPs). These plans, which allow the consumer to pick any participating provider, typically pay hospitals and practitioners on an undiscounted FFS basis. But for most major clinical decisions—such as elective admission to the hospital, nonemergency surgery, psychotherapy, or physical therapy—the practitioner must verify in advance, on pain of nonpayment, that the patient's case meets the insurer's criteria. Some believe that all FFS insurance plans will soon have similar provisions, but as of 1988 MIPs probably represent something less than 20 percent of all private insurance plans. These plans can be considered a third major type of alternative delivery system.

Table 9 shows the probable effect of the major types of health insurance plans on the use of services by patients.

An advertisement from the pages of *Hospitals* seeking institutions to join an integrated "managed care" network.

Table 9 **Probable Effects of Type of Health Insurance Plan on the Delivery of Medical Care**

Characteristic of medical care	Conventional fee-for-service insurance plan	Managed indemnity plan	Preferred provider organization	IPA/network-model HMO	Staff/group-model HMO
Ability to choose primary care physician	+ +	?	–	–	– –
Preventive visits	– –	– –	+	+ +	+ +
Illness-related visits to primary care physician	–	–	+	+ +	+ +
Visits to specialists	+ +	+	+	–	–
Use of diagnostic tests	+ +	–	–	–	–
Rate of surgery	+ +	–	–	–	–
Admission to hospital	+ +	–	–	–	–

Key: Expected impact of plan on consumer use/physician practice (all else equal): – – should decrease, – tends to decrease, ? direction of effect not clear, + tends to increase, + + should increase.

The Shift Toward Ambulatory Care

Largely because payers have found that keeping enrollees out of the hospital saves them money, ambulatory facilities have grown tremendously. As recently as a decade ago, health insurance policies typically excluded ambulatory coverage in favor of the same services provided in hospitals, and patients also seemed to prefer in-hospital care. Today both insurers and patients show a preference for outpatient services. "Some have suggested that patients increasingly associate hospitals with death" (Moxley 1984, p. 196); and this may in fact be a realistic attitude as in-hospital services become increasingly restricted to major surgery and the treatment of major illnesses.

Ambulatory surgery is one newly favored type of medical care now that technological improvements have made it increasingly feasible. Such improvements include better surgical techniques; the use of lasers, which minimize cutting and blood loss; and improved anesthetic agents that "can keep patients asleep for 30 minutes to nearly 12 hours and still leave them clear enough to go home shortly after awakening" (ibid., p. 195). An estimated 40 percent of surgical procedures can now be safely performed in ambulatory settings. Savings have been estimated at 50 to 60 percent per procedure, owing primarily to the elimination of charges associated with the overnight hospital stay.

Since there is no requirement that ambulatory surgery take place out of hospital, many hospitals have responded by setting up their own ambulatory surgery facilities. The patient enters early on the day of surgery, and leaves later that same day. Additionally, there are now independent ambulatory surgery centers (or "surgi-centers") that compete directly with hospitals. In 1987 there were over 500 such facilities, and by 1990 there are expected to be over 1,200.

Other new types of facilities are freestanding emergency-care centers (FECs), urgent-care centers, and convenience-care centers. Offering less expensive care with great accessibility, these facilities were designed to compete with both hospital emergency rooms and conventional doctors' offices. Those using the word "emergency" in their name (often on a neon marquee) must meet strict regulatory requirements: they must be equipped to provide the same care available in a hospital emergency room. There are not many true FECs in the United States. Those that do exist are usually satellite facilities linked to hospitals, and usually provide 24-hour care seven days a week. Many have been built to skirt one or another regulation that applies to hospitals.

Centers not designed to treat critically ill patients are designated urgent-care (or "urgi-care") centers. These facilities are commonly open seven days a week for twelve to sixteen hours a day. Most are equipped to do some laboratory testing and radiological work, and thus to provide episodic care for routine conditions such as sore throats and minor emergencies such as lacerations, sprains, and simple fractures. Many patients view urgi-centers as a backup source of care when their family doctor is unavailable.

Because urgent-care centers charge less than hospital emergency rooms, payers have created reimbursement incentives to encourage their use. This helps explain the recent proliferation of "doc in the boxes" along the major thoroughfares of American suburbs. Unlike hospitals, these centers do not maintain expensive standby equipment and personnel; seriously ill patients are simply transferred to hospitals that can treat them. As a result, urgent-care centers have lower overhead costs and can offer their services at lower prices than hospitals. Some hospitals, in order to maintain their market share, have responded by opening their own lower-priced urgi-centers adjacent to their emergency rooms.

Many urgent-care centers now also offer nonurgent, continuing-care services, creating what have been called convenience-care centers. Commonly located in shopping centers and malls, these facilities attract many patients with their convenience of access. As a further development along the same lines, it is reported that some of the nation's largest retailers are considering offering medical care in their stores, following the earlier success of in-store dental care and optometric facilities.

All told, it is estimated that there were over 2,500 FECs, urgent-care centers, and convenience-care facilities in 1987. This number could easily double by 1990.

Access, 1980s-Style

"Doctors will have to begin appreciating our business and striving to keep it. They'll have to descend to earth." So wrote Jean Lawrence in the *Washington Post* in 1984, pointing up the increasing importance of price, accessibility, and convenience to the patient-physician relationship. In the 1960s the term "access" denoted the need to make care available to the poor and the underserved. In the 1980s it just as often refers to patients' desire for decreased waiting time and lower costs. Lawrence goes on to say, "You [consumers] have a right not to wait more than 15 minutes in the doctor's office."

Effective practice management has become very important to physicians both because patients are demanding convenience and because lower reimbursement necessitates efficiency. Not only have many physicians computerized their record-keeping, billing, and scheduling of appointments, but more and more of them are using marketing services and advertising to attract new patients. Some have gone even further and turned to business management consultants and management-oriented journals in an effort to develop skills that will help them in the competition for patients.

Home Care

Home care for certain kinds of illness is another increasingly popular way of saving money. For many years, agencies have provided chronically ill and infirm elderly patients with hygiene and physical therapy in their own homes as a cost-effective alternative to institutional care; and with the aging of the U.S. population we can expect the number of patients who require this level of care to increase exponentially. But today's technological sophistication has now made it possible to treat additional conditions at home, and technology-based services have added another dimension to home health care.

One of the most significant advances along these lines is portable equipment for intravenous (IV) therapy, which makes it possible to administer antibiotics, chemotherapy, or parenteral

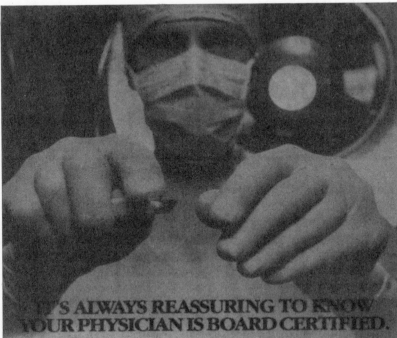

nutrition in the patient's home. Outpatient IV therapy was first reported in the medical literature in 1974. Not only is it less expensive than inpatient IV therapy, but its rate of complications (such as line infection) has been found to be less than or at worst equal to the inpatient rate, particularly at hospitals lacking a full-time IV therapy team. Savings can be significant for conditions such as osteomyelitis, endocarditis, and cellulitis, which all require long-term IV antibiotic therapy.

As expected, payers have perceived the advantages of home health care in such circumstances, and most commercial insurance plans now include home health benefits. Some insurers still pay only 80 percent of home health charges while covering 100 percent of inpatient services, but this policy is expected to change.

Although home health care is covered by most state Medicaid programs, Medicare pays for only a fraction of such services. Even so the use of home health care by Medicare enrollees has increased; the program's expenditures for home care have risen dramatically since 1971, reaching approximately $8 billion in 1985. Both consumers and providers have urged Congress to increase Medicare's home care coverage.

In response to increasing demand and changes in hospital financing, the market for home health care blossomed around 1983. There are now some 6,000 home health agencies of various sizes, with approximately 70,000 home care providers in all. Many hospitals are vertically integrating into the market, and some insurance plans are expected to incorporate preferred home health programs on the PPO model. Also pointed to as a growth area are other nursing home alternatives, such as supported housing for the infirm elderly and adult day care.

Effects of Cost Control Measures

The era of cost control has apparently slowed health care price inflation. *Hospital costs increased only 5.3 percent from 1983 to 1984, compared to an average annual increase of 15.7 percent from 1975 to 1983.* However, per-day costs increased more than 13 percent from 1983 to 1984, indicating that the overall decrease came largely from a decline in days of care.

One factor contributing to increased per-day costs is that end-of-stay days have been largely eliminated; the shorter hospital stay is therefore more resource-intensive. In addition, the percentage of more seriously ill hospital patients has increased now that healthier people are so often treated as outpatients; and of course serious illnesses require more intensive and hence more costly care.

In 1984 health care spending increased less than 3 percent in real terms (adjusted for inflation), the smallest increase in twenty years. However, overall expenditures have continued their steady increase since then (by about 4 percent a year in real terms and 8 percent in dollar amounts), reaching an estimated $497 billion in 1987; and they continue to constitute a significant portion of national spending. How long such increases can go on is not clear. For one thing, a law passed in 1986 requires that the federal budget be balanced by 1991; and decreases in government health spending—some estimate by as much as 2 percent annually—will undoubtedly be part of any balancing process. Moreover, private employer groups are attacking their health care costs with renewed fervor; in 1988 corporate health insurance premium increases (20 percent, on average) were higher than for any other year in recent memory.

In sum, it appears that the new medical marketplace is many things. It is a *vehicle* for cost control, in that many market innovations have been made for that specific reason. It is also a *response* to cost-cutting initiatives, a way of making them work. But it is more than just a vehicle or a response: it has taken on a life of its own. There is no returning to the fee-for-service and laissez-faire days of the 1960s. The revolution has occurred, and the new medical marketplace is not only established but self-perpetuating.

PART II

CARE, COST, AND CONSCIENCE

Ideas are clean. . . . I can take them out and look at
them, they fit in books, they lead me down that narrow way. . . . Ideas are straight—
But the world is round, and a messy mortal is my
friend.
Come walk with me in the mud. . . .

Hugh Prather

CHAPTER 9

THE PHYSICIAN AS ETHICIST

Medical practice takes place in the context of our complex society, in which the health care system is but one element; the goals of the practitioner, of society at large, and of the health care system are not always concordant. The following chapters will examine the most important of the relationships between medical professionals and other participants in the U.S. health care system.

As Dag Hammarskjöld, former Secretary General of the United Nations, once wrote: "You can only hope to find a lasting solution to a conflict if you have learned to see the other objectively, but, at the same time, to experience his difficulties subjectively" (1980, p. 114). In Part I the difficulties in question were those confronting payers and policymakers, and our effort was to make these difficulties and concerns as clear as possible to our intended reader, the medical practitioner. In Part II we turn the focus around and examine the doctor's difficulties and concerns.

Opening Part II with Hugh Prather's poem serves as both a warning and an invitation. The warning is that the waters you are about to enter are murky. Many of the issues examined are controversial, and some will strike close to home. Complex intellectual and ethical questions abound, most with no clear answer that we can see. Yet even if there is nothing to do but muddle on, a map of the terrain is helpful. What we offer, then, is an invitation to enter the waters. . . .

Responsible to the Patient, Profession, or Payer?

For the last three decades there has been a distinct division of responsibility between those who paid for health care and those who provided it. Private insurers and government paid essentially whatever providers charged, in effect endorsing a more-is-better approach to health care. Medical schools taught that practitioners should be accountable only to the patient and themselves—an attitude sanctioned by the population at large. *Society, financing mechanisms, and professional tradition thus mutually reinforced and perpetuated the autonomy of the practicing physician.*

Most physicians, for their part, were insensitive to the cost consequences of their clinical decisions. Few even knew the per-day rates of hospitals to which they admitted patients, or the costs of common diagnostic and therapeutic procedures; and few indeed were conversant with the workings of their patients' insurance policies. Even today not enough physicians are sensitive to these aspects of medical practice.

In effect, the physician was responsible for the care and conscience of medicine, while the payer was responsible for its costs. Since most providers fared well financially under this arrangement, not many were motivated to question it. Table 10 shows that physicians are more satisfied with the system than other key participants.

As we have seen, inefficient medical practices, inflation, and other factors ultimately increased costs to the point where cost containment measures came to seem imperative not only to payers but to society at large. At first, cost reduction measures focused primarily on the hospital; but they have now expanded to include individual practitioners.

To the extent that payers and policymakers have been successful in their efforts to this end, today's physician must not only balance clinical acumen, cost concerns, and conscience, but do so under the scrutiny of powerful third parties to whom costs are *the* issue. Not many physicians enjoy this balancing act, especially in such an atmosphere. *Yet the profession as a whole, and the physician as an individual, have a stake in making the new system work, and thus a duty to speak up while it is still in a state of flux.*

The first step is to clearly identify the desired objectives of payers, consumers, and providers. The second step is for society, with physicians' assistance, to accept and prioritize these objectives or to reject them. It is not only pointless but counterproductive for physicians to resist accommodation to the new era,

Table 10 **Overall Views of the American Health Care System Held by Physicians and Others, 1983**

Answer	500 physicians	100 hospital administrators	1,501 members of the public
On the whole the health care system works pretty well, and only minor changes are necessary to make it work better	48%	41%	21%
There are some good things in our health care system, but fundamental changes are needed to make it work better	48	56	50
The American health care system has so much wrong with it that we need to completely rebuild it	3	2	25

Sources: Louis Harris and Associates 1983, 1984.

since the interest of all parties is best served by their full participation. Also, because some of today's problems were created by practitioners, it can be argued that responsibility for solving these problems rests primarily with the profession.

As Edmund Pellegrino, a noted ethicist and physician, stated in a lecture, medical practice is more than the application of biological knowledge to the diagnosis and treatment of disease: "The heart of medicine is a moral enterprise." Arnold Relman agrees that what physicians are facing "is basically an internal moral crisis" (1983, p. 19).

Physicians, after all, *are inherently no different from other citizens. They have the same strengths and weaknesses of character and are susceptible to the same economic temptations as anyone else. What gives physicians special influence is the trust reposed in them by the public and the responsibility for the care of their patients invested in them by law. This trust and responsibility, in turn, are based on the assumption that the medical profession has unique technical compe-*

tence, which it is committed to employ primarily for the benefit of the sick" (Relman 1985, p. 104).

An exploration of the relationship between the physician as an individual, the profession as a whole, and the medical code of ethics will help us better understand the factors that contribute, both explicitly and implicitly, to the "conscience" of today's provider. A good place to start is the Hippocratic Oath, which all physicians swear to uphold upon graduation from medical school.

Physicians abiding by the Hippocratic Oath have made a formal covenant with patients to do their best for them: this is the intent of the ethic. The principle underlying this intent, known as beneficence, possesses the following characteristics: sympathy, or concern over a person's state of well-being; non-maleficence, or refusal to do intentional harm; and utility, or a sensitivity to the balance between the costs and benefits that may result from one's actions. The physician's beneficence must be balanced by the patient's autonomy: his or her right to have the maximum possible attention paid to what he or she desires.

How well is the intent of the Hippocratic Oath upheld? Pretty well on the whole, most people think, though the centuries-old Hellenic oath has had to be modified in some ways to conform to modern times. For example, its current U.S. avatar, the AMA Code of Ethics, no longer proscribes abortion, and many believe that someday it may no longer proscribe euthanasia. But the evolution of the AMA Code itself raises questions about what is "ethical." If codes, responding to society-at-large, can change over time, *is* there a core of belief at the heart of the medical ethic?

Some physicians might argue that since they themselves are ethical, medical ethics as a subject of study may be left to academic philosophers. But values are one thing, behavior another. A physician with unimpeachable values and morals may still behave unethically by making a clinical decision that ignores a patient's wishes. Medical ethics are not solely an academic matter. They are, and should be, increasingly a matter of discussion at the patient's bedside.

Several key factors affect physicians' decisions. Physicians bring

THE HIPPOCRATIC OATH

I swear by Apollo Physician and Asclepius and Hygieia and Panaceia and all the gods and goddesses, making them my witnesses, that I will fulfill according to my ability and judgment this oath and this covenant:

To hold him who has taught me this art as equal to my parents and to live my life in partnership with him, and if he is in need of money to give him a share of mine, and to regard his offspring as equal to my brothers in male lineage and to teach them this art—if they desire to learn it—without fee and covenant; to give a share of precepts and oral instruction and all the other learning to my sons and to the sons of him who has instructed me and to pupils who have signed the covenant and have taken an oath according to the medical law, but to no one else. I will apply dietetic measures for the benefit of the sick according to my ability and judgment; I will keep them from harm and injustice.

I will neither give a deadly drug to anybody if asked for it, nor will I make a suggestion to this effect. Similarly I will not give to a woman an abortive remedy. In purity and holiness I will guard my life and my art. I will not use the knife, not even on sufferers from stone, but will withdraw in favor of such men as are engaged in this work.

Whatever houses I may visit, I will come for the benefit of the sick, remaining free of all intentional injustice, of all mischief and in particular of sexual relations with both female and male persons, be they free or slaves.

What I may see or hear in the course of the treatment or even outside of the treatment in regard to the life of men, which on no account one must spread abroad, I will keep to myself, holding such things shameful to be spoken about.

If I fulfill this oath and do not violate it, may it be granted to me to enjoy life and art, being honored with fame among all men for all time to come; if I transgress it and swear falsely, may the opposite of all this be my lot.

their individuality to the profession, and to some degree interpret moral behavior uniquely. They bring also their medical training, which inherently implies, as Relman points out, the responsibility to apply it ethically, and in particular an acquaintance with the rules collectively established by the medical profession. In their professional life they are subject to a certain ongoing ethical tutelage, both from peer pressures and from new rulings of the AMA and specialty societies.

Until recently these standards have come only from the practitioner's individual conscience or from the profession as a whole. Today, by contrast, there are additional rules, rules that originate from other sources and have in common an emphasis on financial cost. To accommodate these new rules, some aspects of the professional ethic must evolve and others must be preserved intact. Something we cannot as yet describe is the impact of the professional conscience on the marketplace. The impact of the new medical marketplace on the professional conscience, as well as on standards of care, is described in the next chapter.

CHAPTER 10

BALANCING COST WITH CARE

As the person responsible for most decisions about the use of health care resources by patients, the physician serves as the link between the patient and the medical marketplace. This unique role, which requires both professional and personal judgment, is the crux of the patient-physician relationship. In this chapter we examine how cost reduction requirements are affecting this role.

Entrepreneurialism in Health Care

As we have seen, the increased importance attached to the "bottom line" in health care has been accompanied by a growing competition for both patients and dollars. Management expertise has now become necessary for financial survival. Some entrepreneurial physicians have taken to marketing—a classic demand-inducing strategy—despite doubts in some quarters about whether drumming up trade in this way will lead to improved care for the consumer. Others are raising capital to build facilities that they will then own and operate, and still others are key investors in existing for-profit enterprises.

Owing to the physician's role as the patient's agent, the balance between professionalism and entrepreneurialism is a delicate one. Moreover, because the interests of investor and patient may not always coincide, the arrangement is complicated further if the physician is also an investor in the care facility.

Both patients and health care providers now worry that profit motives are excessively influencing their more entrepreneurial colleagues, to the point of reducing their dedication to patients' needs. The problem is not only ethical but to some extent political. According to Relman, "the medical profession would be in a

stronger position, and its voice would carry more moral authority with the public and the government, if it adopted the principle that practicing physicians should derive no financial benefit
from the health-care market except from their own professional
services" (1980, p. 967).

Yet a respectable argument can also be made the other way,
namely that a physician who invests in a medical facility has more
influence in its operation and can use this influence to improve
the balance between care and cost. Since it is probably easier for
a physician to get a good grasp of cost issues than for a nonphysician manager or entrepreneur to understand medical issues,
physician managers are arguably the better qualified to strike the
right balance.

On a more practical level, the financial solvency of many physicians depends on their investment in for-profit arrangements;
and so, despite Relman's misgivings, such investments will not
be repudiated or disappear. The important thing is that they be
used, so far as possible, to assure that patients' needs remain
paramount.

Practitioners as Employees

Physicians today are perceived by many large for-profit and nonprofit health care organizations as outside contractors or employees: organizational resources rather than independent professionals. In some states (notably trend-setting California) over 50
percent of all physicians contract with one or more HMOs or
PPOs, usually signing papers that give payers certain kinds of
authority over their clinical judgment. Such organizations are
said to "manage" care, a reassuring term to corporate employers
purchasing coverage because it implies a significant ability to control costs. Some anticipate that future physicians may undergo
a "corporate socialization" (Ludmerer 1985) to bring their practice into line with company policy.

Many physicians are in fact employees of others, and their
number is increasing. *About half of all active U.S. physicians now
earn at least part of their income as salary, with many group practices
paying partners by this method.* A continued shift toward salaried
and employee status will be facilitated by the health manpower

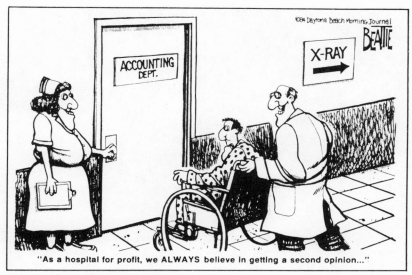

"As a hospital for profit, we ALWAYS believe in getting a second opinion..."

Courtesy of Bruce Beattie and Copley News Service.

surplus, which has reduced both the availability of jobs and physicians' bargaining leverage.

Although there are definite benefits to salaried practice (above all, guaranteed income and scheduled working hours), there are serious drawbacks as well. *Traditionally a fiercely independent group, physicians by and large would rather call their own shots, set their own hours, choose their own patients, shape their own practice; in short, they do not like to be "managed."* For better or worse, the business atmosphere of the health care industry discourages this kind of independence. Another untraditional development, still too recent to assess, is unionization for the purpose of collective bargaining. In 1988 it is estimated that over 40,000 physicians belong to unions, and the number is growing.

Providing Care under Prospective Payment

Under Medicare's DRG-based Prospective Payment System (PPS), most hospitals are now paid a lump sum for the care of each Medicare patient, the amount determined by the patient's primary discharge diagnosis, procedures performed, and age. This

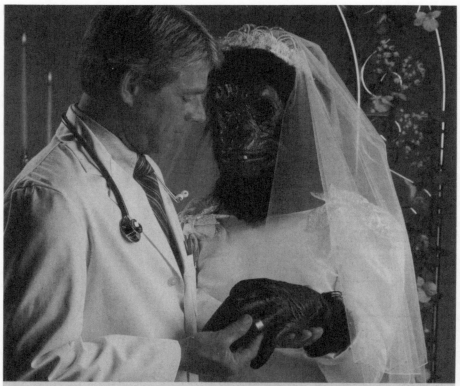

If You've Made An Unholy HMO Alliance, Perhaps We Can Help.

All across the country, physicians who once had visions of a beautiful marriage to an HMO have discovered that the honeymoon is over.

Instead of quality care and a fiscally sound patient-base, they end up accepting reduced fees and increased risks. Plus a lot of new rules that make it more like administrating than practicing medicine.

And while you're doing a lot of the administration, the HMO is charging administrative fees in the neighborhood of 17% to 20%. Small wonder, these HMOs continue to reward distant shareholders with record returns while participating physicians get nothing but grief.

Most doctors have felt there's little or no hope—that "we're trapped" with no way out. But that's not true. There are alternatives. And we're in the business of providing them.

At Prepaid Medical Management Inc., we help physicians develop their own HMOs, negotiate with hostile HMOs or leave contractual situations that have turned sour. And we've been doing it for seven years. In the process, we've helped a number of physician groups profitably leave contracts with national HMOs and establish locally controlled plans with solid fiscal track records.

If you'd like to discuss the alternatives available to your group or IPA, give PreMed President Ed Petras a call. It's not too late to do something about an unholy alliance.

PREMED®

An advertisement from the pages of the AMA's *American Medical News*.

reimbursement change has had a major impact on in-hospital medical care.

There are many ways to profit under PPS reimbursement. One is to decrease labor costs, which account for over 70 percent of the average hospital's budget, by reducing staff-to-patient ratios; many hospitals have done this. Another is to reduce the amount of diagnostic laboratory work performed. Before PPS the diagnostic laboratory was a "profit center" for most hospitals; by inflating charges for tests relative to their costs, hospitals could subsidize other services such as emergency room visits. Under PPS diagnostic tests are no longer a major source of profit. In fact, the reverse is true: the fewer the tests ordered, the larger the hospital's profit.

Another way hospitals can increase revenue under PPS is to encourage physicians to readmit a patient for a second procedure that could have been provided during a prior admission. When this happens a hospital is paid twice for what previously would have been a single hospitalization. Still another strategy, termed "DRG creep," is to place patients into more lucrative categories by making it appear that they are sicker than they actually are; this can be done by reordering, or modifying, the listing of the patient's discharge diagnoses and procedures in the medical record. The hospital administration and financing journals are replete with advertisements by firms guaranteeing that their computer software can improve DRG reimbursements by x percent or y dollars by just this sort of modification.

There is still another way to increase profits under PPS, namely by discriminating—sometimes subtly—among patients based on their medical condition. By sending severely ill patients (or "DRG losers") to other, often municipally owned hospitals, facilities avoid caring for patients who are potentially unprofitable.

Regulatory bodies such as federally sponsored Peer Review Organizations (PROs) attempt to monitor hospitals for readmissions, DRG creep, and inappropriate transfers, all of which work against the intent of PPS by raising costs. But the PROs' task is difficult: *no payment system is completely immune to manipulation intended to benefit those providing the service.*

Although most facilities are earning profits under PPS, provi-

An advertisement from the pages of the *Journal of Health Care Financial Management.*

ders are critical of several aspects of this payment approach. Payment under PPS is based on *average* resource use and length of stay, but patients who are severely ill consume more resources than average. Severity of illness is affected by whether or not there is an accompanying condition, the timeliness with which patients seek care, complications such as drug reactions, and many other factors beyond the control of the provider. Yet PPS reimbursement does not allow for payment increases for more severely ill patients unless complications put them into another DRG or their treatment reaches the outlier cutoff, at which point the hospital is paid on a cost basis. *Since hospitals lose money on severely ill patients under PPS, their incentive is to treat only the least severely ill and to discharge patients after the minimal length of stay.*

Another difficulty with PPS is its basis in DRGs, many of which have been called by their critics "Damn-Ridiculous Groups." For example, Guillain-Barre Syndrome, with an average length of stay of 40 days, is categorized in the same DRG as migraine headache, which rarely requires hospitalization. Most components of severity of illness are not accounted for under the present DRG categorization scheme, though this defect will likely be remedied by one or another of a variety of "severity of illness" methodologies now being tested.

Providers and policymakers have other worries about PPS reimbursement. Under the FFS system, which encourages the use of tests, treatments, and procedures, patients are theoretically at risk for too much care. Under PPS, by contrast, in which more care results in fewer "excess revenue" dollars, patients are at risk for receiving less care than they require. The same thing is true of HMOs, since HMO providers benefit, at least in part, from any profits made by the plan when revenues exceed expenditures. *Under either DRGs or capitation, practitioners derive economic rewards from providing less care.*

Another disadvantage of the new system is that it gives short shrift to the intangible rewards of patient care. As Mitchell Rabkin pointed out in 1982, prior to the implementation of PPS, the early days of hospitalization are anxious ones for both the patient and the provider. The patient is sick; the provider is working to diagnose the condition and initiate treatment. In contrast, the last days of the hospital stay are relatively gratifying, as therapy takes effect and the patient's condition improves. Under the new system patients leave the hospital just as the days of gratification begin. The physician loses both ways: the overall intensity of in-hospital care increases, and there is no balancing gratification from observing the patient's return to health.

As a consequence of decreasing length of stay, hospital workloads have increased and the general atmosphere of most hospitals has become more emotionally intense and anxious. These changes have severely affected the hospital's front-line professional, the floor nurse, leading to a critical exodus of nurses who find their workloads have increased drastically while their compensation has not. House officers have been affected as well. Needless to say, these changes put added strains on the patient-provider relationship.

The Changing Hospital-Physician Relationship

Although to date PPS has most directly affected hospital management, it has also indirectly affected physicians by changing their working arrangement with hospitals. Hospitals are no longer merely workshops for practitioners; today hospital administrators are actively involved not only with monitoring physicians' practice in terms of cost efficiency, but with actively urging them to use preadmission testing, order fewer expensive diagnostic tests, perform fewer procedures, and discharge patients earlier. Physicians may also be asked to increase the number of admissions they make to the hospital. Computer systems are now commonly used to calculate the average length of stay by DRG of patients admitted to the hospital by individual physicians or aggregate staff, and to assess these averages against a hospital-selected standard. Most institutions monitor such cost and resource use data for their staff physicians; few take into account clinical outcomes such as morbidity or death rates.

Some hospitals now grant practice privileges partly on the basis of economic performance, thus putting a premium on cost efficiency in locations where gaining such privileges is no easy matter. Other hospitals now contract directly with practitioners to care for patients, choosing their specialists carefully with an eye to maximizing profits. Such facilities may especially favor family practitioners, whose services are generally less expensive than specialists'. More and more hospitals now also grant privileges to non-M.D. providers such as dentists, podiatrists, and midwives as a way of increasing their total patient load.

Relations between hospitals and their medical staffs are sometimes strained by the fact that whereas hospitals receive PPS reimbursement, most physicians (as of 1988) are still reimbursed by FFS. Some hospitals have tried to compensate for the differing sets of incentives under Medicare's PPS and CPR reimbursements by introducing penalty or reward systems to make physicians more cost-efficient. Others have initiated "joint venture" corporations, such as the Medical Staff and Hospital (MeSH) arrangement discussed in Chapter 8, whereby the institution and its staff share any PPS profits. One critic believes that "the conflict inherent in joint ventures is far more insidious [than in FFS payment]. Here the unethical physicians would garner extra revenue, not from recommending that which is not needed, but from *not* recommending that which *is* needed. Here the tool is silence, rather than persuasion. And patients may never realize that potentially beneficial options are being denied to them. They are thus poorly situated even to consider obtaining another opinion" (Morreim 1985, p. 35).

Effects of Cost Controls on Education and Research

Another casualty of PPS reimbursement is medical education. The new system has had particularly acute effects on university teaching hospitals, not only because they are centers to which the severely ill patients are referred, but because the "extra" educational and research tasks they perform make them less cost-efficient.

When initiated in 1983, PPS allowed for a "graduate medical education add-on" to teaching hospitals amounting to 11.56 percent of the total reimbursement per DRG. As of 1987, this add-on had been reduced to 8.7 percent, significantly decreasing the revenues of teaching hospitals. Furthermore, other third-party payers seem likely to follow Medicare's lead and reduce the portion of their reimbursements that subsidizes residency training programs. The issue of how (and whether) payers should reimburse hospitals for their training activities is the subject of considerable debate.

PPS has also helped to erect barriers against the application of new technologies, particularly those that improve care without also improving cost efficiency. PPS reimbursement regulations currently include an annual increase for purchasing new equipment, but this increase is significantly lower than the usual increase before DRGs. As a result, the financial ability of most hospitals to introduce technical improvements has decreased.

Another problem is the lack of an adequate DRG for patients

admitted to the hospital under experimental protocols. Outlier dollars are supposed to subsidize the care of patients participating in research studies, but these funds are inadequate even for the care of severely ill patients, and protocol patients tend to be still more expensive. To solve this problem, it has been proposed that a new DRG be added expressly for such patients.

The strained financial situation experienced by teaching hospitals has been further exacerbated by increased competition for patients and the shift toward for-profit health care. For-profit multihospital systems typically select favorable markets for development, such as the Sunbelt region, where they find less regulation, charge instead of cost reimbursement formulas, and an expanding and comparatively affluent population. As a result, urban academic medical centers often are left to care for the poor and the most severely ill. Moreover, for-profit hospitals avoid becoming heavily involved in education, with its high overhead costs. In a health care industry that is increasingly price-competitive, teaching hospitals risk being squeezed out of the market.

Managing Physicians' Decisions

As we have seen, payers and policymakers have an increasing say in practitioners' medical decisions. From the cost perspective this makes sense: payers, including government, benefit when costs are kept down. From the care perspective, however, it makes considerably less sense. *The clinical decision-making process is, and always will be, replete with uncertainty.* Because utilization review alone is inadequate, professional judgment must remain a key component in this process. *Moreover, the outcomes of many decisions can affect patients profoundly; and the ultimate responsibility for these decisions, from both an ethical and a legal perspective, rests with the physician, not the payer or policymaker.*

Physicians are in effect caught in the middle. They are simultaneously responsible on the one hand for meeting societal and managerial cost control objectives, and on the other for the welfare of patients who desire improved health essentially without concern for costs. Indeed, the current system seems to be moving practitioners inexorably in the direction of making explicit trade-offs between cost and quality.

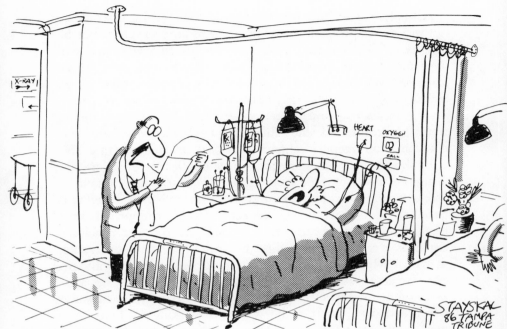

"YOUR BLOOD PRESSURE AND TEMPERATURE ARE WAY UP, BUT YOUR MEDICARE COVERAGE IS WAY DOWN. LOOKS AS IF YOU CAN GO HOME TODAY, MRS. FITCH!"

"The burden of proof about activities in medicine is shifting so that the presumption is no longer that what the physician chooses to do is automatically correct and must be proven wrong. Rather, increasingly the burden of the physician is to justify why he should perform in a 'higher-cost' manner if it does not offer substantial and worthwhile benefit to the patient" (Fineberg 1985, p. 37).

In the era of cost control, third parties have displayed a new distrust of health care providers, whom many see as having abused their autonomy, privilege, and power over the last twenty years or more. Providers argue that if their charges decrease, the quality of care will decrease. But payers have empirical data showing that costs can be cut considerably without decreasing quality, and they conclude that the real concern of the provider lies elsewhere. What is *really* at stake, they ask: the care of the patient or the income and status of the physician?

Actually, net income for physicians is decreasing if we define net income as professional compensation after expenses but before taxes. *AMA data for 1983, for the first time in many years, showed a 3 percent overall income decline in real terms from the year before, probably owing chiefly to lower reimbursement levels, an increasing supply of young physicians competing for patients, and a greater number of practitioners on fixed salaries.* In general this trend has continued since then, but payers would plainly welcome an even steeper decline as part of their effort to cut costs.

In short, payers and providers have conflicting goals and differing perspectives. One would not expect providers to willingly accept fewer dollars and growth restrictions, which is in fact what payers want. Nor would one expect payers to willingly pay more for services that they can get for less and that they see as being of equal or even superior quality. The resulting "zero-sum game," in which whatever one side wins the other loses, has hindered effective action toward reasonable compromises.

As might be expected, patients are also becoming increasingly concerned with whether the system is working to their advantage, or whether (like poor Mrs. Fitch in the cartoon) they are mere pawns in some financial chess game. *Today's patients may come to feel they have no true advocate within the health care system.* There is no easy answer here. Patients now have more say in decisions made about their care, and will probably have even more in the future. But tradeoffs will have to occur because even with the patient as Priority 1, societal objectives will exact their due.

The Inevitable Tradeoff

The assumption behind many of today's cost control measures is that waste can be removed from the system while necessary services are retained. As a result of such measures, fewer new dollars (in adjusted per capita terms) are now entering the health care sector, and the idea is to spend these dollars first on what is truly necessary. In theory these reduced funds will be sufficient if the 25 percent or so of all care now deemed unnecessary is trimmed from the system.

Like most such formulations, this one is deceptively simple, assuming as it does the ability to identify which services are necessary and which are excessive. It is hardly possible to "trim the fat without cutting into the meat" when there is no agreement on what is fat and what is meat. In these circumstances tradeoffs have inevitably been made, many of them uncritically.

It will never be easy to balance resource constraints against the patient's best interest, but the process *can* be made more rational. The following chapter explores the strengths and deficiencies of the medical decision-making process in the present era.

CHAPTER 11

MAKING CLINICAL DECISIONS

Clinical decision-making is the process used to determine whether a test or treatment should be ordered or performed, given a specific constellation of patient signs, symptoms, and social circumstances. Observed practice patterns represent the outcome of such decisions. For example, when a child has a third pharyngeal beta strep infection within a twelve-month period, will a physician refer that child to a surgeon for tonsillectomy? Will an internist order a chest x-ray automatically for every patient he or she admits to the hospital?

One of the earliest studies of practice pattern variation was carried out in the 1930s with a group of 1,000 eleven-year-olds in New York City. Of this group, 65 percent had already had their tonsils removed. Those with tonsils intact were examined by a group of physicians, who recommended tonsillectomy for 45 percent of them. Those for whom it was not recommended were sent for examination by another group of physicians—and 46 percent of *them* were selected as candidates for tonsillectomy. When this process was repeated again for the remaining children, tonsillectomy was advised for a comparable percentage. At this point only 65 children remained for whom tonsillectomy had not been recommended, and "the study was halted for lack of physicians" (Eddy 1984, p. 84).

The practice patterns within a population of physicians (or of patients they treat) can be ascertained by geographically oriented "small-area variation" studies. According to a landmark work of this type carried out by Wennberg and Gittelsohn: "In one area of Vermont the tonsillectomy rate from 1969 through 1971 was such that if it had persisted, 60 percent of all children would have had their tonsils removed by age 20. In a second Vermont area the rate was such that only 8 percent would have had their tonsils removed by age 20" (Wennberg 1982, p. 121). As another example,

Medicare data since 1966 consistently show hospital length of stay for given conditions to be 2.5 days greater in the Northeast than in the West, with the South falling between these two extremes.

Similar results have been found in both cross-regional and international studies. Some surgical procedures, including hysterectomies, tonsillectomies, and prostatectomies, have consistently shown high variation (up to sixfold) across populations or regions; others, including cholecystectomies, appendectomies, and hernia repairs, show low variation (often less than threefold). Significant variations have also been shown in the treatment of several medical conditions.

Why this happens is not at all clear; attempts to explain small-area variations by differences between patient populations in age, sex, race, and severity of illness have not been completely successful. Nor is it clear which rates represent the "best" level of care. *But one thing is certain: by its very nature, wide variability indicates that some patients are receiving suboptimal care. It also undercuts the position of those practitioners who believe they should be left entirely on their own to make decisions, free of guidelines or oversight. Finally, it supports to some extent payers' contention that some practice patterns cost too much and that costs can be reduced by identifying efficient practice patterns and adequate (but not excessive) levels of care.*

The Role of Uncertainty

One reason clinical decision-making varies so widely is the role that uncertainty plays in this process. Physicians are frequently uncertain whether a disease is present, whether a particular diagnosis is right, what diagnostic tests or procedures to prescribe, and what treatment is most appropriate in terms of anticipated outcome, patient consent, and compliance. Physicians vary in their tolerance for uncertainty as well and, as Figure 12 shows, in their willingness to discuss their uncertainty with patients.

Probability theory offers one way of reducing uncertainty in responding to a given set of diagnostic test results and patient characteristics. In particular, Bayes' theorem of conditional probability can be used to subject the new data and all relevant prior quantitative knowledge regarding the patient to known pat-

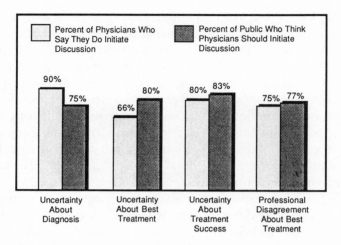

Fig. 12. Uncertainty in medical care and the physician-patient interaction. (Source: President's Commission for the Study of Ethical Problems in Medicine and Biomedical and Behavioral Research 1982.)

terns of probability. For example, based on a patient's age, sex, and history, S-T wave changes on electrocardiograms have a very different (and predictable) likelihood of reflecting arteriosclerosis. By using Bayes' theorem (or a computer program based on it) a physician can readily plan the best course of diagnostic testing for a specific patient, based on the state of the literature at the time. Few physicians as yet are comfortable with this approach, however. Most prefer to rely on their training, experience, and intuition.

Ordering tests is a common way to reduce uncertainty, one that has become more common with the proliferation of new tests. *As new tests and treatments are developed, physicians incorporate them into practice, often in an additive rather than integrative manner.* Fuchs (1974) has termed this practice the "technological imperative."

Some economic influences support expensive clinical decisions as well. Under FFS reimbursement, as we know, resolving uncertainty by doing more coincides with the physician's financial incentives. With the growth of malpractice litigation, discussed in the next chapter, defensive medicine has also become a significant influence on decision-making. A third factor is that most patients have insurance coverage. "The Medical Uncertainty Principle states that there is always one more thing that might be done—another consultation, a new drug, a different treatment. Uncertainty is resolved by doing more: the patient asks for more, the doctor orders more. The patient's simple rule for resolving uncertainty is to seek care up to the level of his insurance" (Walsh 1977, p. 21).

Attempts to resolve uncertainty can have negative consequences. Iatrogenic damage can occur during the diagnostic process, for example, and false-positive test results can lead to inappropriate treatment. In addition, a provider who orders too many tests may be penalized for attempting to decrease uncertainty below the point condoned by payers.

Quality and Waste

To confront the issue of waste in health care, it is necessary to agree on workable definitions of such basic but elusive concepts as "quality" and "waste." Avedis Donabedian, a seminal thinker on the quality of care, defines quality as follows: "At the very least, the quality of technical care consists in the application of medical science and technology in a manner that maximizes its benefits to health without correspondingly increasing its risks. The degree of quality is, therefore, the extent to which the care provided is expected to achieve the most favorable balance of risks and benefits" (1980, p. 4).

Excessive diagnostic testing is a good example of waste. Up to a certain point, the information derived from testing contributes to the quality of care. Eventually, however, the knowledge obtained from additional tests will provide no useful information. At some point the risks or costs of testing outweigh its benefits, and at that point the downward turn in the quality curve begins. Waste also increases costs. As Donabedian writes: "Quality costs money, but it is possible by cutting out useless services and by producing services more efficiently to obtain higher quality for the money than is now spent on care, or to have the same quality at lower cost" (ibid., p. 7).

From the perspective of cost *or* quality, then, decreasing waste is desirable. But waste is not easily identified: test results are not returned from the lab labeled useful, useless, or questionable. We need some alternative way of defining where waste begins, and perhaps the logical place to begin is with the economist's concept of marginal benefits. Economists conceptualize an ideal system in which the cost of the latest unit produced (the marginal cost) equals the price consumers are willing to pay for it (the marginal price). Something like this theoretical point is where clinicians should begin the process of trimming waste: eliminating care that costs more than it is worth.

For example, the American Cancer Society recommends that six guaiac exams be performed annually on all people over age 40. This series of tests would detect approximately 93 percent of all asymptomatic colon cancers. But an analysis of this practice estimated that "the marginal cost of the sixth test—\$47.1 million per cancer case detected—was 20,000 times the average cost per case discovered" (Estaugh 1981, p. 33). The question that payers and policymakers have asked all along, and that the profession is now beginning to ask itself, is this: "Although six sequential stool guaiacs, followed by barium enemas for all positive guaiacs, will identify virtually all asymptomatic colon cancers, is it worth \$47.1 million to detect that one rare case when the resources could be used elsewhere?" (ibid., p. 33).

Many more analyses of this sort are needed before we can be reasonably sure that the money spent on health care is being spent in the best possible way. At the moment, we lack not only the information such studies would give us but also an institutionalized or system-wide method for allocating the resources entering the health care system. Physicians in effect find themselves making decisions that society by rights should make. The economist Uwe Reinhardt describes the difficulty of this task:

"While detached policy analysts may find it easy to discourse upon the value of life from a safe distance, no one has yet given the individual physician a publicly sanctioned set of guidelines under which to make cost-quality trade-offs at the patient's bedside. So far, society has delicately preferred to leave that matter to the physician's own judgment. . . . The providers of health care must reckon with the prospect that society will increasingly both flagellate them over health care costs

and saddle them with ethical dilemmas no politician (and possibly not even most economists) would have the courage to face in the trenches" (1985, p. 57C).

Technology and Uncertainty

Another source of uncertainty is how to apply medical science and technology. All too often, new medical technologies are applied before their cost, safety, and usefulness are adequately considered. Indeed, some analysts believe that new medical technologies are proliferating beyond the profession's capacity for assessing them properly. It is a fact, for example, that very few treatment modalities (new or otherwise) have been subjected to randomized clinical trials. As a result, "Often in medical practice . . . 'the right thing' is simply a matter of opinion because many tests, procedures, and operations have not yet been fully evaluated or scientifically compared with other available measures for cost effectiveness" (Relman 1985, p. 105).

Moreover, new developments are usually disseminated through the medical literature, and this is not a value-free process. Authors naturally want to have their work accepted by the profession, and thus their reporting tends to be favorable. Peer review mitigates this tendency, but neither is it an unbiased process. The customary means of reporting adverse effects is the isolated case report, a process that tends to severely underestimate the actual incidence of complications. The result is a medical literature that is probably undercritical of new developments.

As an example, the Swan-Ganz catheter was favorably reported in the literature and information about its use spread quickly and informally among clinicians. Its benefits are undeniable in appropriate clinical circumstances, but complications can and do occur. Why? At what rate? We don't really know. Even though the Swan-Ganz catheter is widely used, it has yet to be fully evaluated in clinical trials. In short, even though its use "has assumed epidemic proportions" (Robin 1985, p. 445), it may or may not be helpful to a given patient or class of patients.

An opposite problem is a strong attachment to the current accepted practice even when the superiority of a newer practice can be clearly demonstrated. Staying with the known element, with its known properties, seems safer than taking the risks that accompany change; yet the costs resulting from such inertia can be high. An example is the use of screening chest x-rays:

> The practice of ordering chest films to screen patients admitted to hospitals gained popularity after World War II, when tuberculosis was prevalent in this country. Early studies indicated that twice as many cases of tuberculosis were found among patients screened on admission as among those screened in a mass outpatient survey. However, as the prevalence of tuberculosis decreased, so did the prevalence of abnormalities detected on the chest x-ray film obtained on admission. Later, physicians began to use chest films to screen for lung cancer, hoping that with early detection, more patients would be cured. Several large studies have shown no significant difference in mortality rates between patients in whom lung cancer is detected by chest-film screening and those in whom the disease is detected by other methods, and the American Cancer Society no longer recommends chest-film screening for this disease. (Hubbell 1985, p. 212)

Many practitioners used to ordering admission chest x-rays have resisted abandoning this practice. It is estimated that more than $1 billion is spent annually in the United States for routine preadmission chest x-rays. And this is but one of many costly tests that are overused or used in an outmoded style.

Yet things seem to be improving. With the stress on keeping costs down by using technology efficiently, the "technological imperative" is exerting less influence than it once did. Rather, biomedical science is being guided more and more by "technology assessment" or "medical practice evaluation." Such practices have had a particularly dramatic effect on reducing the time patients spend in the hospital. For example, over recent years average time in the hospital following coronary artery bypass surgery was decreased from twelve days to seven with no adverse effect on recovery.

Two quantitative approaches used to assess treatment alternatives are cost-benefit analysis and cost-effectiveness analysis. In a cost-benefit analysis (CBA), a monetary value is assigned to both inputs and outcomes—for example, a year of life saved, or a year made more productive—in an effort to determine which of two or more alternative health care services, each with very different

Government poster encouraging workers to seek a chest x-ray, circa 1940.
(Source: University of Minnesota Libraries, Social Welfare History Archives.)

impacts on society, is to be preferred. CBA, for example, might be used to decide whether to allocate resources to a cancer screening program or a coronary care unit.

In a cost-effectiveness analysis (CEA), no assignment of monetary value is made to outcomes and the effects are measured in nonfinancial units such as years of life saved or morbidity avoided. Since different outcomes are not translated to a common denominator, CEA can only be used to compare programs or treatments with similar effects: for example, treatment of coronary occlusion with surgical intervention vs. medical management.

Protocols for Decision-Making

More than ever, physicians are cooperating with epidemiologists and health service researchers in efforts to develop practice protocols. Technology assessment, clinical trials, and research on outcomes of care all provide information that can be used together with the results of small-area variation studies to create new empirically based "standards" of care.

As Morreim says, "One cannot practice good medicine by committee or cookbook or computer" (1985, p. 34), but computers can help. In one project, researchers used mathematical modeling to develop "Clinical Prediction Rules" based on observed probabilities and clinical experience. In such a system the patient's symptoms are entered into a computer, which estimates the probability that the symptoms are indicative of a particular disease. One system of this sort has been helpful in determining how to treat patients with pharyngitis (such as whether or not to prescribe antibiotics).

A more conventional role for computers in medicine is in record-keeping and information processing. Computerized medical information systems have been used effectively in a number of hospitals and outpatient settings, and in some of them this information retrieval capability has been linked with limited treatment or diagnosis-assistance capabilities as described above. This dual application, including routinized computer-based reminders, can only help improve both the quality and the efficiency of medical practice. When the computer's ability to store and process vast amounts of information is added to human judgment, the best of technology can be combined with the best of the healer's art.

Another effort to standardize medical practice is the NIH's Consensus-Development Program. Established in 1977, this program has sponsored over fifty conferences at which leading specialists discuss the state of knowledge, diagnosis, and treatment of major conditions in their specialty.

Protocols of standard practice will increase in importance as more patients move into managed-care systems such as HMOs, where standardization helps administrators control costs and quality. There are advantages from the physician's perspective as well: "[Protocols] provide a basis for encouraging cost conscious behavior on the part of physicians in hospital settings, but they do so by allowing physicians, as a collectively responsible group, to set their own clinical standards, which effectively constitute financial standards as well" (Young 1985, p. 17).

Once fiscally responsible "ideal" standards have been developed, they must be disseminated by specialty societies, hospitals, and other organizations. But even when rationally developed standards are widely disseminated, real change can occur only if the individual practitioner is persuaded to modify his or her practice. Several studies suggest that this will happen: for example, surgery rates decreased in one locale when practitioners learned that their rates fell outside the average range in their area.

Although this approach seems to be a start toward finding an ethical balance of care, cost, and conscience at the bedside, many practitioners understandably see norms of care as a serious threat to their independence. They foresee a day when rote, predetermined plans mandated by payers and hospitals will be ubiquitous or even exclusive approaches to patient care. And indeed some hospitals already place explicit restrictions on physicians' practice, and others use economic incentives to sanction undesired behavior and reward cost efficiency.

Practitioners typically resist this type of control, perceiving it as an insult to their professionalism. Perhaps more palatable than administrative fiat is the peer group approach, where approval or sanction comes from a group of peers or clinical superiors. Any such approach, however, must be truly responsive to the cost concerns of managers and payers; and this has not always been the case in the past.

Scientifically derived standards for care have not yet been developed for many conditions, in part because of difficulties at both the scientific and political levels. In their absence most payers will continued to use "low users" as their point of reference, arguing that high users should conform unless they can make a strong case to the contrary. Physicians can only respond by doing what is best for their patients, given the resources available. At times this may mean agreeing with payers that less is sufficient; but at other times it may mean standing firm and insisting that more is necessary.

Guidelines for Efficient Use of the Hospital

There are other, simpler ways to decrease costs and increase efficiency while maintaining quality. Some commonsense principles for hospital care have been suggested by seasoned, efficient physicians that would go a long way toward reducing unnecessary medical care. The following practices, surprisingly, are not followed in a significant proportion of cases:

- Be certain that the patient requires admission by assuring that the services needed cannot be provided outside of hospital.
- If the patient needs treatment, do it as early in the course of an illness as possible.
- Do as many tests as possible before admission.
- Do not admit patients electively on a Thursday or Friday if they require tests or procedures that are not available on weekends.
- Do not admit patients electively for surgery unless operating room time is scheduled.
- Make sure that those services ordered (tests, procedures, vital signs) are indicated and are consistent with the provision of proper care.
- Sequence tests and procedures in a timely manner. Become familiar with radiology and laboratory prep protocols (for example, patient preparation for a barium swallow) to avoid delays and assure that the patient gets the most out of a test.
- When a consultation is sought, make sure that the question is well defined and that the consultation is both necessary and timely.

- Begin planning for discharge on the day of admission by considering the degree of home or institutional support the patient will require and by involving the discharge planners sooner rather than later.
- Write discharge orders the night before the expected day of departure, so that patients are able to leave early on that day.
- Document why tests and procedures are being performed. Documentation not only clarifies matters for other physicians and nurses, but is used by utilization reviewers and payers for reimbursement and quality assurance purposes.

Guidelines for Ordering Diagnostic Tests

Despite the difficulty of developing protocols for ordering tests, some practical guidance can be given. There are several important things to know about any diagnostic test, notably its risk, accuracy, interobserver variability (particularly important for x-rays and electrocardiograms), patient acceptability, cost, and utility compared to other diagnostic modalities. When ordering or performing a specific test or procedure, a physician should consider the following questions:

- Will the test really provide useful information that will affect the care of the patient? If so, will the result be timely and will someone use it?
- Is the test part of a routine protocol that has been passed down over the years and needs to be reevaluated? Would another test yield better information?
- Is a test being ordered quickly ("stat") because speed is medically necessary or will decrease the patient's length of stay and charges, or is it just to have a number for rounds? When a large percentage of chemistry and hematology tests are ordered stat, not only are charges higher but it makes the term meaningless, since the laboratory staff cannot know which tests are actually needed right away and should be given priority.
- Last but not least, would the test or procedure be ordered if the physician had to carry it out personally, or pay for it, or had to take it himself or herself or have a close relative take it? This is really just another version of the Golden Rule.

Future Directions

As new approaches to decision-making become more prevalent, the role of biomedical ethics will increase in importance. While physicians work toward incorporating economic considerations in their practice, beneficence, patient autonomy, and justice must remain central to the patient care process.

In an environment characterized by strong incentives to minimize care, physicians increasingly find themselves arguing with third-party payers over the existence of extenuating circumstances for patient X's hospitalization or over patient Y's need for a specific type of care. Unwelcome as such arguments are, making them is now part of the role and responsibility of the modern practitioner as the patient's agent. At times, if necessary, the physician may have to accept lower reimbursement—or even no reimbursement—for providing the care that is deemed to be in the patient's best interest. Whatever the temptations to the contrary, now more than ever each major clinical decision should be arrived at by careful analysis and not by rote.

Medical education will be an important means of gaining the profession's acceptance of new methods of clinical decision-making. Traditionally medical education has generated a "rule-out mentality," a disposition to order every conceivable test in an effort to rule out a range of diseases. This has also been described as "the 'roundsmanship mentality,' wherein one is criticized for not having ordered the serum cauliflower test" (Tobin 1980, p. 288).

Attitudes must change. The incorporation of computers, protocols, practice evaluation, and other innovations by didactic role models is now critical to learning effective medical practice. Students who see Bayes' theorem and a "rule-in" mentality applied in clinical situations will be far more likely to use these strategies themselves. By adopting a fiscally responsible and efficient decision-making style, preceptors will prepare students and house staff for the decisions they will be called on to make in today's medical marketplace.

CHAPTER 12

THE MALPRACTICE CRISIS

Medical malpractice is faulty medical management that injures a patient. Plaintiffs must prove fault on the part of a physician, hospital or other provider of care, recognize damage to themselves, and a causal connection between the two. Almost always, fault consists of negligence" (Bovbjerg 1985, p. 38).

Malpractice occurs and tort law* is breached if a physician injures a patient through practice that is not up to acceptable standards. Those found guilty of malpractice may be required to make good any economic damages resulting from the injury, and in many states additional money may be awarded for pain and suffering. Providers purchase medical malpractice insurance against the possibility that they will be sued for large sums.

The Malpractice Crisis

Most would agree that compensation is due a patient who has been harmed by a physician's mistake. But difficult questions of definition and degree are involved in determining that compensation, and these questions have broad ramifications not only in medical practice but throughout society. In recent years a variety of factors—including the structure of the legal system, social attitudes, changes in health care financing, and uncertainty in clinical practice itself—have combined to create a crisis of sorts for the medical profession.

Although the notion of malpractice has roots in medieval

---

* A tort is a legal wrong committed upon the person or property of another for which the law gives civil remedy, usually monetary damages for the resulting injury. Common torts are negligence, assault, battery, false imprisonment, libel, slander, and invasion of privacy.

times, actual lawsuits against physicians were rare until this century. In the past several decades there has been a steady increase in the number of malpractice suits, and this trend has accelerated in recent years. The AMA reports that prior to 1981 an average of 3.2 claims per 100 physicians were made annually. *Between 1981 and 1984 the rate increased to 8.2 claims per 100 physicians, and in 1985 it reached 10.1 per 100 physicians.*

Although any physician may be sued, certain specialties generate a higher percentage of suits, notably obstetrics and gynecology, general surgery, and orthopedic surgery (see Table 11). In contrast, other clinicians such as family physicians and midwives are sued infrequently.

Not only has the number of suits increased, but judges and juries have increased the amounts awarded to successful claimants. Data from a firm specializing in legal case analysis indicate that the average medically related court award increased from $229,000 in 1975 to $888,000 in 1983, and to over $1,000,000 in 1985. These figures exclude out-of-court settlements.

What kinds of cases are being brought to court? In 1983 the St. Paul Insurance Company, a major malpractice insurer, reported that among its policyholders the most common reasons for being sued were:

- a bad result, such as complications resulting from negligent post-surgical care
- falls of all types, including from bed, while walking, and in the bathroom
- delayed or omitted treatment
- injury of a body part adjacent to the treatment site
- wrong diagnosis or incorrect treatment
- infection, contamination, or exposure to an injurious substance

Uncertainty, Errors, and Expectations

The attribution of error is fundamental to the determination that medical malpractice has occurred. The Latin phrase *res ipsa loquitur,* "the thing speaks for itself," is used in some states when an

Table 11 **Average Incidence of Malpractice Claims by Specialty, 1985**

Category	Annual claims per 100 physicians
All physicians[a]	10.1
Specialty:	
General/Family Practice	5.5
Internal Medicine	6.3
Surgery	16.5
Pediatrics	7.6
Obstetrics/Gynecology	26.6
Radiology	12.9
Psychiatry	2.4
Anesthesiology	6.5

Source: AMA 1986, p. 13.
[a] Includes physicians in specialties not listed separately.

error is so obvious that no further explanation of it is necessary; the classic example is the proverbial "Kelly in the belly."* The argument that medicine is an inexact science is irrelevant if the provider has made such an egregious error.

As medical technologies advance, however, it becomes harder to distinguish between a poor outcome resulting from negligence or error and a poor outcome resulting from natural events. As a consequence, many lawsuits brought against physicians today do not involve their negligence but result from events and outcomes largely beyond their control. One serious problem is that doctors and lawyers have different standards of evidence. "Scientific evidence must be probable, repeatable, provable. Legal evidence needs merely to be possible, sometimes only remotely possible. Large liability awards for scientifically unprovable but legally possible injuries following alleged acts of malpractice or negligence have become commonplace" (Lee 1986, p. 159).

Uncertainty is inherent in medicine: not only uncertainty about the condition of a particular patient, but uncertainty about

---

*A Kelly is a type of surgical clamp. This phrase was coined to refer to an x-ray revealing a surgical clamp remaining in a patient's abdomen after the surgery was completed and the incision closed. The phrase is now used to refer more generally to such obvious mistakes.

the "best" course of treatment. Even experts frequently disagree. For example, two articles in the same issue of the *New England Journal of Medicine* came to conflicting conclusions on the extent to which postmenopausal women increased their risk of cardiovascular disease by using estrogen (Stempfer 1985; Wilson 1985). Some physicians today are being sued because bad outcomes resulted from reasonable and unavoidable differences in opinion about medical practice.

Some blame the malpractice crisis on a sharp increase in the actual commission of malpractice by practitioners. They contend that only a small percentage of the increasing number of injuries caused by physicians' errors ever result in lawsuits; and the fact that so many suits are settled out of court does imply, if not that the provider was guilty, at least that the insurance company considered the circumstances unfavorable for a solid defense. On the other hand, many cases are dismissed in pretrial hearings because they lack merit; and in cases that do eventually reach the courtroom, plaintiffs are awarded damages less than half the time.

Furthermore, if an increase in the actual occurrence of malpractice is causing an increased number of lawsuits, one would expect a few doctors to be sued repeatedly. In fact, lawsuits are widely dispersed: some 60 percent of obstetricians, for example, have been sued at least once in their careers. Table 12 shows the percentage of physicians, overall and by specialty, who have been sued at least once.

The patient-physician relationship has played a role in malpractice. Many patients believe that there is "always" a drug, device, or treatment to cure any condition. Practitioners reinforce this misconception to some extent, and a paternalistic bedside manner may reinforce it further. The danger is that if the patient is then *not* cured, or has a less than ideal outcome, it seems logical to blame the physician for negligence or error. *Indeed, the idea has arisen that financial compensation is due when there is a bad outcome, whether or not it resulted from a physician's error.* Increasingly tort law is seen simply as a system to provide compensation for injury, and malpractice suits have evolved into a type of lottery where a big win is possible.

In the United States an initial dollar outlay is not required to

Table 12 **Physicians' Experience of
Lawsuits by Specialty, 1985**

Category	Percent of physicians sued at least once during their career
All physicians[a]	36.5%
Specialty:	
General/Family Practice	34.4
Internal Medicine	28.7
Surgery	49.5
Pediatrics	27.7
Obstetrics/Gynecology	64.0
Radiology	38.8
Psychiatry	15.8
Anesthesiology	35.6

Source: AMA 1986, p. 14.
[a] Includes physicians in specialties not listed separately.

bring suit. Most malpractice lawyers' fees are paid as a percentage of the amount awarded, known as a contingency fee. In Great Britain, by contrast, citizens must pay a lawyer's fee in advance to file a lawsuit, and a claimant who loses a suit must pay the defendant's legal costs. For this reason, among others, there are far fewer malpractice suits per capita in Great Britain, and malpractice insurance premiums are accordingly much lower.

Medical Malpractice Insurance

The medical malpractice insurance industry, which for years had been a safe and lucrative business, became financially unpredictable in the mid-1970s with the sharp increase in the number and amounts of awards. Panic led several major companies to withdraw from the market, leaving many providers without protection. "A few others remained, but raised their rates dramatically, in some states by as much as 300 percent in one year. Physicians were faced with the choice of paying exorbitant premiums, 'going bare,' finding other sources of coverage, or limiting or quitting their practice" (Williams 1985, p. 1). Practitioners who "go bare" do not purchase malpractice insurance; if they are sued and lose, they pay the damages out of pocket.

After some insurance companies withdrew from the malpractice business, some practitioners could not find policies at any price. And when those malpractice insurers who remained increased their prices sharply, as much as 500 percent for some specialists, many could not afford the new premiums and were forced to "go bare." Some states responded to the crisis by limiting the amount of awards. And some for the first time permitted groups of physicians or medical societies to found their own malpractice insurance companies, known in some quarters as "bedpan mutuals."

Today, premium prices vary widely, depending on specialty, geographic area, and other factors. For instance, a neurosurgeon in New York City pays much higher premiums than a psychiatrist in the rural midwest. Because of these wide variations, data can be presented selectively to support the argument that malpractice premiums are not becoming unaffordable. Indeed, aggregate data indicate that premium payments have remained stable over the past ten years at approximately 4 percent of the average physician's yearly gross income (see Table 13), which is not a staggeringly high percentage.

But selective and aggregate figures hide the truth. A crisis of insurance affordability has in fact occurred, especially for specialists such as neurosurgeons and obstetricians. In 1985 U.S. obstetricians paid an average malpractice insurance premium of $23,300; for many the amount was much higher. In Maryland the *average* was $42,000. Some New York City neurosurgeons are now paying more than $100,000 annually for malpractice coverage.

The traditional malpractice insurance policy is the "occurrence" type, which covers care provided during the coverage year. Thus coverage in 1978 would insure the purchaser against all lawsuits involving incidents of that year, even a suit filed ten years later.

In an effort to lower prices, many companies have now shifted to a new kind of policy that insures only against suits *filed* during the year for which payment is made. Under such a policy, the physician who pays malpractice premiums in 1988 has purchased insurance only against lawsuits filed that same year. Because suits

Table 13   **Average Annual Professional Liability Insurance Premiums of Self-Employed Physicians by Specialty, 1985**

Category	Average premium
All physicians[a]	$10,500
Specialty:	
General/Family Practice	6,700
Internal Medicine	5,800
Surgery	16,600
Pediatrics	4,700
Obstetrics/Gynecology	23,300
Radiology	9,100
Psychiatry	2,600
Anesthesiology	18,000

Source: AMA 1986, p. 16.
[a] Includes physicians in specialties not listed separately.

are often filed years after an incident occurs, this coverage is far more limited than an occurrence policy. It is less expensive, but the dollars spent buy less protection. Although some physicians would rather pay more for the extra protection afforded by an occurrence policy, many companies no longer offer this type of policy.

Effects of the Malpractice Crisis

The malpractice crisis has changed the way medicine is practiced. It has led to "defensive medicine," the attitude that a practitioner had better provide every possible service because if the patient's outcome is less than ideal the practitioner might be sued for negligence. Physicians with this attitude, and there are many, order more tests, refer patients to specialists earlier and more often, and perform fewer high-risk procedures.

Obstetricians are now much more likely to refer high-risk patients to tertiary care referral centers, and the incidence of Cesarean sections is increasing to the point where in 1987 it was estimated that 100,000 unnecessary C-sections a year were being performed. Both of these phenomena are due in part to the increased fear of complications and subsequent litigation. Malpractice itself has become one of the most common complications;

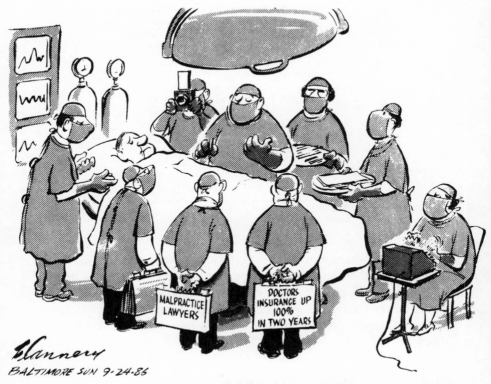

BALTIMORE SUN 9-24-86

"Scalpel. . . Legal Pad. . . Pencil. . ."

some obstetricians fear that any child born less than perfect may become the subject of a lawsuit.

A defensive practice style may lead to the discarding of certain harmful procedures, but its disadvantages are many. Because virtually all diagnostic tests carry inherent risks, extensive testing increases the possibility of iatrogenic disease. Moreover, patients and their insurers must pay for the extra tests, and these problems escalate as more tests and treatments become available.

The threat of malpractice has also made an impact on the patient-practitioner relationship. People have become more distrustful of the care they receive; there is even a service available in some cities for patients to check a practitioner's lawsuit record.

Wary patients are less open to a physician's recommendations and reassurances, dampening the positive effects that a clinical encounter should produce.

Practitioners, too, have become wary, and in some cities subscribe to a new service that offers notice of patients who sue frequently. Many physicians have also become cynical toward the legal system, whose premises they see as unrealistic.

"For practitioners of liability litigation, a utopian medical world in which all illness is preventable or discoverable and curable by brilliantly empathetic and encyclopedic physicians is indispensable. [They] have created a biologic bill of rights predicated on the notion that illness and injury are unnatural and therefore somebody else's fault. In this non-Darwinian world, the biology of the individual is susceptible only to the actions of other human agents" (Lee 1986, p. 159).

The malpractice crisis also has significant consequences for society as a whole. First, taxpayers must support an expensive legal system to process these lawsuits. Second, malpractice insurance premium costs are said to account for 2 percent of the dollars spent on health care, since most such costs are passed along to patients and payers in the form of higher charges. *Even more important in cost terms are the indirect effects of defensive medicine.* From *12 to 25 percent* of the increase in health care costs has been attributed to altered practice patterns. Estimates vary, but it appears that some $15-$40 billion annually is spent on defensive, and otherwise unnecessary, medical care.

As we have seen, payers are no longer willing to make reimbursements for care meant primarily to benefit the physician, which means that the present high rate of expenditure on medically marginal or unnecessary services cannot be sustained. As reimbursement is ratcheted down, practitioners will no longer have the option of practicing defensive medicine; indeed, prepaid and capitated plans actually penalize such behavior. Yet the physician remains liable for complications resulting from early discharge or tests omitted to save money. Small wonder that today's practitioner "naturally feels caught between the lawyer and the hospital administrator" (Siden 1986, p. 523).

The availability of medical care is also affected by the high cost of malpractice insurance. Physicians whose expenses are higher

because of expensive malpractice premiums are less ready to treat
indigent patients; and other inner-city patients are also affected
because young physicians prefer to establish practices in geographic locations with lower premiums. Medical graduates are
now reluctant to train in high-risk specialties such as obstetrics
and neurosurgery. And many obstetrician-gynecologists are simply eliminating the obstetric component of their practice; some
25 percent of those located in Florida now limit their practice to
gynecology. For all these reasons, decreased access to some types
of medical care has reached crisis proportions in some areas.

Dealing with the Malpractice Crisis

There are several possible ways of dealing with the malpractice
crisis. One of the most promising is tort reform legislation. More
than two hundred organizations have joined together to form
ATRA, the American Tort Reform Association. The formation
of ATRA was initiated by groups of bus drivers, teachers, manufacturers, sports teams, and others who today must pay expensive malpractice premiums because of the high risk that they will
be sued in the course of offering their services to the public. Physicians have joined with these groups to lobby for reform.

It is estimated that only 28 to 40 cents of every premium dollar
goes to the victims of malpractice; the rest goes to insurance
companies and lawyers. Elected federal and state officials could
do much to minimize the malpractice crisis by passing laws that
would change these proportions.

A number of tort reforms have been proposed in an effort to
deter claimants from bringing nonmeritorious suits. For example, some states permit countersuits. When the option of
countersuit is available to the defendant, persons without valid
suits are less likely to sue.

Several different types of awards are made to claimants who
win malpractice suits. "Compensatory" damages are meant to
replace the patient's economic losses. "Punitive" damages are
meant to punish defendants found guilty of willful malpractice.
Some states have abolished punitive damages, arguing that they
punish only the insurance company and that there are more effec-

tive ways to punish delinquent physicians. "Pain and suffering" awards are meant to compensate the claimant for the emotional damage caused by the malpractice. Some states place no financial limit on such awards. Others do limit them on the argument that doing so makes patients and their lawyers less likely to file a doubtful suit.

Another proposed tort reform is designed to ensure that expert witnesses-for-hire (who provide services to both sides of the case) truly are expert in their fields, so that judges and juries can base their decisions on the most accurate testimony possible. Still another reform, which has been adopted by some states, is reducing the length of time after an incident during which a person can bring suit (known as the statute of limitations). With a decreased amount of time available to file, the number of lawsuits is reduced.

Many other types of tort reform have been proposed, among them a no-fault system. By 1987 more than 35 states had passed laws designed to limit malpractice awards and claims. A number of states have not passed any laws to date, and reform has been incomplete in many others; but people in the health care industry are generally encouraged by what is happening.

Tort reform alone, however, will not solve the malpractice problem. Changes must also be made within the medical profession. For one thing, stringent quality assurance programs should be developed to improve the overall quality of medical care. Also, as discussed earlier, developing norms of care to assist the decision-making process would not only improve the quality of care, but also, by eliminating some of the gray areas of practice where uncertainty and vulnerability are highest, decrease the risk of suits in those areas.

It has been suggested that "legal standards" of practice be formulated as a way to support practitioners' arguments in court. Currently states have different standards of malfeasance for practitioners' actions. Some states judge such actions by the local standard of care, but in other states lawyers have successfully argued that given the extent of modern communication through the media as well as the medical literature, physicians should be held liable if they fail to provide the best care currently available anywhere in the country (or the world). Lawyers and others working in the court litigation process support the development of uniform standards of care. Evidence that a practitioner has adhered to accepted standards always helps the defense.

Yet caution must be exercised in using uniform standards of care as courtroom evidence. Each medical case is unique. Human judgment not only cannot be replaced by protocols, but is indispensable in deciding whether or not a protocol applies to a given case. The danger of uniform standards is that they might be used to convict a physician who made a perfectly appropriate decision not to follow a protocol. By contrast, there is significant ambiguity in tort law definitions, with much leeway for interpretation by the court, so that each case may be examined on its own merits.

Internal policing and disciplinary actions by physicians are important aspects of the solution to the malpractice crisis. *The number of practitioners who are censured or have their licenses revoked by state medical societies is astoundingly low.* Peer review must be strengthened, and protected from antitrust lawsuits. Stiffer regulations regarding relicensing and improved continuing education programs are also needed. Such initiatives would diminish the force behind many lawsuits, since then "the public would not regard the courts as the only safeguard against incompetent physicians" (Angell 1985, p. 1207).

While these changes in the system are being made, there are several things the individual provider can do to minimize the risk of a malpractice suit. One is to keep abreast of new medical developments. Another is to seek help when it is needed. Still another is to involve patients increasingly in decisions regarding their own treatment, being frank with them about the uncertainty of outcome in medical care. Patients and family members who participate in a decision will be less quick to challenge it in court, and less likely to succeed if they do.

Another useful move, and one that costs little or nothing, is to be more courteous to patients. Appointments should be scheduled such that a patient's waiting time is kept to a minimum. Office personnel should be given instruction in telephone answering technique, and in the importance of respecting the patient's desire for courtesy and privacy in the office and the examining room. Even modest improvements along these lines can do much to reduce the frustration many patients feel in their interactions with the health care system. They have also been shown to reduce the incidence of lawsuits.

Complete, up-to-date medical records are another asset in today's litigious atmosphere. Not only is an accurate record of a patient's visits, tests, and treatments critical to good medical practice, but it can serve as a valuable aid to memory in the event of a malpractice suit. It also provides physical evidence of the practitioner's perspective and actions. For all these reasons, physicians should not alter or allow staff members to alter records. Any necessary changes in the chart should be initialed and dated; deletions should be made in such a way that the deleted words can still be read. Details of how informed consent was obtained should be documented in a particularly careful fashion, and the major points covered in the discussion with the patient and family should be included. Only well-accepted abbreviations should be used. Dictations should be read before they are signed. Lastly, records should be kept indefinitely: computers and microfilm save space.

Poor outcomes and mistakes cannot be entirely prevented. But the current atmosphere of extreme litigiousness, mutual distrust, and extravagant dollar awards, even in cases where physicians acted competently and in good faith, should be corrected. Such improvements would benefit patients, physicians, medical care, the justice system, and society as a whole.

CHAPTER 13

ENSURING ACCESS TO HEALTH CARE

As priorities regarding health care delivery change, the care of poor and underinsured patients has resurfaced as one of today's most critical health policy issues. The main problem is cost. Although the "poor" are covered by the federal-state Medicaid program, there is also a sizable group of "near-poor," people whose income is low by most standards but not low enough to qualify them for Medicaid. Persons in this category, whose numbers are growing substantially as support for government programs is reduced, are usually unable to afford either health insurance premiums or medical bills.

Another class of disadvantaged persons are those with disabilities or major illnesses. Not only do such persons face significant impediments to employment and therefore to eligibility for employer-sponsored health benefits, but their condition may make it impossible for them to purchase commercial insurance protection.

In 1987 it was estimated that 15 percent of all Americans, or about 37 million persons, had no health insurance. This group is primarily composed of the "gray area" near-poor below age 65, children, those unable to purchase coverage because of disability, unemployed persons, and persons whose employers do not offer health insurance benefits.

U.S. Policy Toward Medical Care for the Poor

A century ago the poor were treated in charity hospitals; many paid nothing for their care. In later years government assumed increasing responsibility for care of the poor, and various social welfare programs were introduced. In the mid-1960s government policymakers attempted to assume full responsibility for the health care of the poor by introducing Medicaid, and access to care by poor Americans improved considerably as a direct result of this program. Table 14 shows that income no longer determines quantity of medical services received; compare the obviously income-related disparities in dental care, which is not fully covered by public-sector programs.

Making medical care more accessible to the underprivileged unquestionably helped to improve the health of the U.S. population. Thus, whereas the infant mortality rate remained essentially unchanged in the decade preceding the introduction of the Medicaid program, in the next fourteen years it decreased from 25 to 13 deaths per 1,000 live births. Death rates for "poverty-related illnesses," such as maternal mortality, influenza, pneumonia, gastrointestinal diseases, and diabetes, also declined significantly after Medicaid began (Davis 1985). On a societal level, the average life expectancy of the U.S. population rose steadily from the turn of the century until the mid-1950s, when it leveled off. It began rising again in the late 1960s following the introduction of Medicaid.

The relationship between dollars spent on health care and improved health is not necessarily one-to-one: other factors, such as nutritional programs and pollution control, have a positive impact on health. *Nevertheless, the data clearly show that such public spending does improve health by increasing people's use of medical services.*

In the 1970s and early 1980s changes in U.S. health policy in response to economic pressures resulted in decreased public subsidies to health care. Some states did not cut Medicaid spending, but simply tried to hold their program budget constant; this was a common approach for local health programs as well. However, because of price inflation both in and out of the health care sector, a constant level of funding effectively meant an 8–10 percent decrease in real spending.

Government policy got tougher in the 1980s. The Reagan Administration "called for major cutbacks in entitlement to health care for the poor and elderly" (Davis 1985, p. 51); and although some of the more drastic proposals were modified or rejected by Congress, reductions were still made. Another result of this

Table 14 **Physician and Dentist Visits and Hospital Discharges and Episodes, by Race and Family Income, 1983**

Race/ethnicity and family income	Physician visits		Dentist visits		Hospital episodes	
	Number per person per year	Percent of persons with 1 or more visits	Number per person per year	Percent of persons with 1 or more visits	Average discharges per person per year	Average days in hospital per episode
Total	5.0	74.0%	1.8	51.8%	1.3	6.7
Race:						
White	5.1	74.4	1.9	54.0	1.3	6.5
Black	4.8	73.0	1.2	37.7	1.5	8.2
Income:						
Under $10,000	5.9	73.6	1.2	37.4	1.7	7.7
$10,000–14,999	5.0	71.5	1.4	41.9	1.3	7.0
$15,000–19,999	4.7	73.1	1.6	46.6	1.2	6.4
$20,000–34,999	5.0	75.1	2.2	57.5	1.1	5.8
$35,000 or more	5.4	78.1	2.7	70.4	1.1	6.4

Source: USDHHS 1986.

policy shift was lifting the requirement that public facilities keep records of free care provided to indigent patients and report them as part of their continuing Hill-Burton obligation.

Compared to other publicly funded programs, Medicare and Medicaid have borne a proportionately larger share of the total cuts made by the Reagan Administration. Although expenditures measured in current dollars have continually increased, the increases have fallen behind the rate of inflation, with the result that public-sector support of health care has in fact decreased.

The New Competitive Industry and the Poor

An age-old problem in the health care field, dating from even before the days of pesthouse hospitals and bloodletting, is that physicians and hospitals have difficulty collecting payments once their services have been supplied. After the enactment of social welfare programs such as Medicaid, providers were reimbursed for more of the care that they had previously donated. Because of this, some argue that the health care industry has benefited from these programs as much as the poor over the last several decades.

Yet because public programs have never enrolled 100 percent of those unable to afford services, "uncompensated care" has remained a fiscal issue for health care providers. Until recently this issue has been comparatively insignificant for most hospitals, because the financing system, intentionally or not, included sufficient slack to pay for the uninsured. Hospitals in effect used "extra" dollars collected from patients and payers via "inflated" charges to help cover expenses incurred by charity patients.

But times have changed, and today we have cost containment measures such as prospective payment, capitation, and managed care whose specific goal is to eliminate such practices. With today's price-based competition, payers increasingly negotiate discounts and insist on the reimbursement of costs rather than charges. As a result, discretionary funds available to hospitals for charity care have decreased considerably.

This is more of a problem in not-for-profit hospitals than in for-profit hospitals. Although it appears that investor-owned hospitals and nonprofit hospitals in the same geographic areas provide roughly comparable amounts of charity care, the majority of for-profit hospitals are located in affluent areas where the poor are not close at hand. As a result of their location, then, as well as their for-profit mission and their financial responsibility to investors, they treat a lower proportion of poor people than the nonprofits.

Nor do the poor generally have access to the growing number of independent outpatient facilities. Such facilities, as we have seen, can charge significantly lower prices than hospital emergency rooms for comparable services; but because they are primarily investor-sponsored and not mandated to care for the poor, most require payment (or an insurance card) at the time of service. As a result, the poor are further concentrated in the already crowded emergency rooms of inner-city and public hospitals.

Teaching hospitals, often situated in urban ghettos, have traditionally cared for a large proportion of the poor. In 1982 they reportedly provided nearly half of the free care in this country, although they had only 6 percent of the country's acute-care beds. A law passed in 1985 included a PPS formula to increase payments to hospitals caring for a disproportionate percentage of either the poor or Medicare Part A beneficiaries, the first time such an adjustment had been made. Ironically, however, the new dollars came from funds that would otherwise have gone to support graduate medical education, thereby canceling any gains that teaching hospitals might have realized.

Effects of Cost Control on Care of the Poor

Medicaid has been touted as the health care "safety net" for the poor, but recent policy decisions have poked big holes in the net. Both the absolute number *and* the percentage of the nation's poor covered by Medicaid have fallen. This trend began in the mid-1970s and has continued through the 1980s. In 1980 about 10 percent of all Americans under 65 were uninsured for at least some time during the year; in 1986 an estimated 15 percent of people under 65 were uninsured for the entire year, approximately one-third of them children under seventeen. (See Figure 5, p. 29.) In families below the poverty line, 34 percent of all children have no insurance coverage.

As a result of the shifts in government reimbursement policy, today's system lacks a mechanism to ensure that providers offer their share of charity care. The responsibility has fallen on selected facilities such as teaching hospitals, which, because of the very same trends, are now less able to exercise it. Hospitals that want to go on providing care to the poor often cannot afford to do so.

New reimbursement methods have created additional incentives to transfer the poor to public hospitals. A recent Chicago-based study found that 87 percent of the patients transferred to Cook County Hospital (a public hospital) were sent there primarily because they lacked adequate third-party health coverage. There are more and more reports of women in labor, and heart attack and stabbing victims—some with IV lines in place—arriving on a transfer basis at public hospitals.

Under the old social contract the *cost of indigent care* was the hot potato passed from providers to paying patient. Under the newly emerging contract, the *bodies of the uninsured poor themselves* become the hot potatoes that are being dumped from provider to provider. Politicians ought not to feign surprise at this transformation, nor ought they to remind physicians of the Hippocratic Oath. Indeed, to blame doctors and hospitals for the practice of "patient dumping" all the while refusing to legislate the means of paying for the care rendered to uninsured indigents strikes one as disingenuous. (Reinhardt 1986, p. 8)

Dumping of this sort became especially common in Texas, with its numerous for-profit hospitals, its high unemployment rate, and a Medicaid program ranking 48th in the nation in level of payments. In that state, legislation was recently passed in an effort to stem the flow of indigent patients transferred from private to public facilities. Other states are expected to follow suit.

As a result of inadequate access to medical care, gains in health status made in recent years may be eroding. A California study compared a group of people whose Medicaid coverage had been terminated a year earlier with a control group who had remained in the program. The former group was found to have increased hypertension, higher mortality, less opportunity to obtain care, and less satisfaction with the care received.

Critics have charged that government is retrenching without an explicit private-sector plan to fill the resulting gap. While the negotiations and political maneuvering continue—signs of a system in flux—increasing numbers of indigent people are being left with little or no medical care. Even from a financial perspective, decreasing access to care in this manner makes little sense. People who do not receive timely medical care in the early stages of an illness become seriously ill, and may then require resource-intensive hospitalization. Apart from the numerous ethical questions this raises, neither patient nor payer benefits. Figure 13 shows recent changes in the availability of health care to the poor.

Possible Solutions

If health care is viewed simply as a commodity comparable to any other in the U.S. market, its distribution should be on the basis of ability to pay. If, by contrast, health care is "a social good of special moral importance" (Daniels 1986, p. 1381), society has an obligation to ensure all its members a reasonable level of access to such care.

There are several possible approaches to reform. *One is a universal "national health insurance" program. The United States is the*

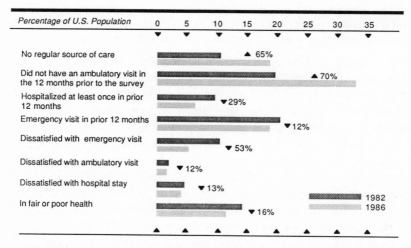

Fig. 13. Changes in access to health care, 1982–1986. (Source: Robert Wood Johnson Foundation 1987.)

only major industrialized nation that has not instituted such a program. Proposals have been made and debated in Congress since the 1930s, but to no avail; the last time such a law was seriously considered was in 1976.

There are several reasons for opposing a national health system. First, there are doubts whether such a system would control costs. Second, U.S. society places a high value on personal choice, and a national health system would of necessity limit the range of choice. Third, and probably most important, the powerful health care provider and private insurance industries vehemently oppose the idea. For these reasons and because of the present political and economic climate, national health insurance legislation is unlikely to be passed in the near future. In the more distant future, however, some analysts think that continued conflicts with numerous unaccountable private payers may lead providers to support a federally based system with its accountable, publicly elected "board of directors." Others believe that the spread of AIDS (a disease whose victims often cost the system well over $100,000 during the course of their illness) will force a unified, nationally sponsored approach to health care financing.

A more limited reform would be to extend Medicaid coverage

to those on the current margins of eligibility (that is, to the near-poor). Some have also suggested joint public-private initiatives to make work-related health insurance available to those marginally employed at part-time or low-level jobs; such employees constitute a large proportion of uninsured Americans. Still another proposal is to retain the arrangement whereby higher charges to insured persons help subsidize care of the uninsured. This type of subsidy arrangement is already in place in some states.

Role for the Healing Professions

Physicians' opinions may (and should) have some influence on the direction and intensity of health care reform. Table 15 shows physicians' attitudes toward some proposed reforms in health care coverage for the unemployed.

In 1980 David Rogers, a former medical school dean and head

Table 15   **500 U.S. Physicians' Attitudes Toward Health Insurance Coverage for the Unemployed**

Proposal	Percent in favor	Percent not in favor
Encouraging but not requiring each state to pay for health care coverage for unemployed workers	69%	28%
Requiring employers, by law, to maintain health insurance benefits for laid-off workers for 6 months and contribute to a pool of funds to provide another 12 months of coverage	62	34
Financing health care coverage for the unemployed by establishing a federal government program similar to the Medicare program	43	54
Establishing a tax on third-party payers to finance extension of benefits for the unemployed	34	62
Financing health care coverage for the unemployed from new taxes on individuals' employer-paid health insurance premiums that exceed a set amount	31	65

Source: Louis Harris and Associates 1984.

of the influential Robert Wood Johnson Foundation, testified before a Congressional subcommittee about the dramatic increase in visits to physicians by the poor and by nonwhites after the establishment of Medicaid. (During the same time period, the number of visits by white and nonpoor persons remained fairly steady at a higher level.) Challenging the behavior of physicians in providing care to the poor, Uwe Reinhardt posed this disquieting question: "Would [one] interpret the sudden upswing in the physician care received by America's poor since the mid-1960s as (a) a massive attack of unrequited noblesse oblige seizing members of [the] profession shortly after 1964, or (b) a sudden decrease in the health status of America's hitherto unusually robust and healthy poor, or (c) the emergence of federal financing of physician care for America's poor, many of whom were sick all along?" (Relman 1986, p. 12).

Although neither the Hippocratic Oath nor the AMA Code explicitly states that practitioners must provide charity care, this sort of moral obligation is part of what sets medicine apart from other professions. With expected privileges such as autonomy and status comes a degree of social responsibility. Precisely what degree is debatable; but to judge from the 1982 bad-debt average for all U.S. general hospitals, a reasonable proportion of hospital revenues designated for charity care appears to be 5 percent annually. Arguably a facility with a percentage significantly lower than this should be more involved in providing such care, and physicians using such a facility should be involved in seeing that this happens.

Physicians can also take the lead in developing formal protocols for the transfer of indigent patients to other facilities. To be sure, motivations for transfer are often mixed: some transfers are clearly mandated on medical grounds. An argument can also be made that the uninsured should be treated predominantly at taxpayer-sponsored facilities. But for once the central issue is simple: the patient's interest and well-being must be the paramount concern. In the words of George Annas, a lawyer and health care ethicist, "Physicians cannot and should not permit themselves to be used as financial hatchet-men by profit-maximizing hospital managers. They should act as conscientious objectors to hospital policies that put patients at risk" (1986, p. 76).

Physicians can also act on their own by providing a certain amount of free or reduced-price care; accepting assignment from Medicare; becoming a Medicaid Participating Physician (which some consider a type of charity service because of low reimbursement levels); giving lower-income patients more time to pay bills before passing them on to a collection agency; and donating time to free clinics and shelters for the homeless that provide medical services.

Charity care is more than an ethical responsibility; it is also a way for practitioners to repay their debt to society. Today public funds pay for most medical research; thus in some sense the resulting knowledge belongs to society, not to the profession. Through taxes society further subsidizes both public *and* private medical education, a subsidy estimated at the substantial amount of $30–$50,000 per year per student. Thus even students paying full tuition receive the majority of their support from public funds. Likewise, residency training is subsidized up to $90,000 per trainee per year with revenue obtained directly from government and third-party payers. Many countries providing similar levels of subsidy require all physicians to provide government service, often of several years' duration, in return. In this country, charity care may be thought to represent the equivalent of such service as an ethical responsibility, a professional obligation, and a way to repay a debt to society.

CHAPTER 14

THE 1990s AND BEYOND

Health care is but one of many sectors of society with a claim on our collective resources. Can we have both bottom-line repair and better health care? Because our wealth is not infinite, priorities must be set; and the main way priorities are set in the United States today is by social and political pressure.

In the face of increasingly stringent cost-containment measures, health care consumers have become politically organized to protect their interests; especially in instances where their positions appear to be at odds with those of providers. (See Table 16). We observe this trend in the growth of organizations such as women's health cooperatives and the transformation of the American Association of Retired Persons into a powerful Congressional lobby for the elderly. "For the first time, health interests have shown signs of forming a broad coalition to battle the administration's budget reductions" (Iglehart 1986, p. 1464). Although such groups generally support today's health care industry, they have pointed to many serious deficiencies in our existing delivery system; and they continue to address tough questions to payers, provider organizations, and the healing professions.

The Human Dimension

Biomedical knowledge has been applied so successfully to the treatment of many major diseases that the process of death and dying has become redefined. Many Americans worry that if they become terminally ill, machines of one sort or another might be used to deny them a dignified natural death. The hospice movement arose in response to this worry. It is clear now that patients' desires are in some cases better served by less intensive care.

Many also ask why the medical profession—as compared, say,

with dentists—has shown only modest interest in activating the patient as a participant in his or her own care. As the hazards of cholesterol, smoking, and alcohol abuse became widely known, many people changed their eating habits, stopped smoking, and cut down on alcohol. The medical profession, while formally advocating and applauding these changes, in actuality did little to promote them. As a result, health-conscious people in the 1970s rarely turned to traditional practitioners for advice or instruction in how to stay healthy.

Table 16 **Acceptability of Proposed Cost-Containment Policies and Programs: Physicians and Public Compared**

Proposal	Proposal very or somewhat acceptable		Proposal not very or not at all acceptable	
	Physicians	Public	Physicians	Public
Requiring employees to pay a part of their health insurance premiums	82%	65%	16%	32%
Requiring patients to pay a greater part than they now pay of all their medical bills covered by their health insurance to encourage them to watch their medical expenses	71	52	27	46
A system that encourages people to have tests and minor surgery done in clinics and doctors' offices rather than in hospitals	93	83	6	16
A system in which the patient has to obtain from the insurance company payment approval for specific expenses and length of hospitalization prior to nonemergency hospitalization	41	57	57	41
In the case of nonemergency surgery, requiring the patient to get a second opinion from another doctor to find out if the surgery is necessary	74	88	23	10

Table 16 (*continued*)

Proposal	Proposal very or somewhat acceptable		Proposal not very or not at all acceptable	
	Physicians	Public	Physicians	Public
A system that discourages a hospital from having expensive equipment and specialists, if they are available at another hospital nearby	65	62	33	36
A system in which the fees paid to doctors and hospitals for treating all patients with particular types of diagnoses are fixed	37	76	61	21
Government price controls of doctors' and hospital fees	13	61	85	36
A health plan where, for a monthly fee paid in advance, you receive physicals, doctors' visits, and hospitalization no matter how often you use these services	40	61	58	36
Including only hospitals and doctors with lower prices in a health insurance plan, and excluding those that are more expensive	34	62	63	34
Limiting the use of expensive medical technology for patients who have virtually no hope of recovery	59	49	37	46

Sources: Louis Harris and Associates 1983, 1984.

Today's physicians are more responsive to the human dimension of medical care than those of twenty years ago; but they have a long way to go. Some feel that a major effort to ascertain, publicize, and diminish life-threatening habits may be the next significant step toward improving the human condition, and most at least concede that physicians can play a significant role *before* pathology occurs. Not that technological intervention has become

Ever Wish You Had A Doctor Who Specialized In You?

Meet The Family Practice Specialist.

Family Practice is the specialty of overall health care for the whole person. Family Physicians specialize in the basic medical needs of each family member — from newborn to grandparent. And that includes you.

From a national advertisement campaign sponsored by the American Academy of Family Physicians.

less important; it is simply that lifestyle is increasingly seen as much more important than it was once thought to be.

Biomedical Research: A Social Priority?

As recently as several decades ago, fear of disease was an everyday experience for most Americans. To raise a family without at least one casualty from a communicable disease was the exception rather than the rule. A childhood victim of polio remembers that "each summer, when the epidemics peaked, public swimming pools, camps, and even churches were closed. Children were kept at home, and victims and their families were shunned by many of their neighbors" (Calmes 1984, p. 1273).

In contrast, most citizens today no longer have a personal terror of disease. With very few exceptions, U.S. children are no longer crippled by polio, scarred by smallpox, or incapacitated by rheumatic fever or tuberculosis. Ironically, one result is that the value formerly placed on medical research has declined; at least that is one way of reading the current all-out emphasis on cutting costs. Some think the AIDS epidemic may reverse this trend, since it has raised fears similar to those once engendered by polio.

Strangely enough, problems that scientists have *not* conquered have had a similar effect on social attitudes. Several common diseases remain largely incurable despite today's technologically sophisticated armamentarium. Some result from habits such as smoking and alcohol abuse, or from social and environmental problems such as violence and industrial hazards. Such conditions have become the bane of modern existence, analogous to infectious diseases in previous eras; and many believe that the medical profession can do little more than treat their victims.

Other chronic diseases of less clear origin seem to be just as incurable in our present state of knowledge. One problem is that the "half-way technologies" used in treating such diseases—for example, dialysis for end-state renal disease and the artificial heart for terminal cardiac disease—are extremely expensive. Expenditures for such high-tech medicine have been blamed as a major cause of the runaway inflation in health care costs, with only modest returns in terms of improving the nation's health.

For all these reasons—high costs, overzealous application,

questionable benefit—some people now are uncertain whether society gets a sufficient return on its investment in biomedical research. Both public support for medical research and actual funds (adjusted for inflation) have decreased, and reductions have been made in both hospital reimbursements and grants to medical school research centers. Some institutions have cut back significantly on research; others have sought private, sometimes proprietary, financing. Many fear that if research funding continues to shift to the private sector, future research efforts will be chosen more for their potential profitability than for their potential impact on society.

The direction of medical research is also being questioned in another way. In an effort to cure such major epidemic diseases as polio, medical research has for many decades been directed toward exploring pathological mechanisms. Some people now feel that this path of inquiry is too narrow, that "the turbulence of relentless scientific analysis needs to be stilled" (O'Day 1984, p. 7) and the basis of investigation broadened to include the social, emotional, and psychological aspects of disease.

Some research projects of this broader sort are under way. Yet any tendency toward increasing the "relevance" of research has its dangers, notably that what seems relevant today may not seem so tomorrow. Conversely, what appears to be an unpromising research project today may become a major breakthrough in disease treatment tomorrow. One thing seems certain: a reasonable level of research is needed if there are to be any breakthroughs at all.

How Should Health Care Resources Be Allocated?

If one accepts the premise that society is responsible for the health of its members, then all members have a right to at least a basic level of care. But how does one determine what is "basic?" Does each citizen have a right to an annual physical exam and preventive health care? To treatment of life-threatening conditions only?

At the societal level, how can our health care resources be used to do the most good? At the individual level, can they be distributed to provide all with an equal opportunity for health? What is the fair thing to do? Alas, views about fairness differ widely; well-intentioned people favor different courses of action in a given situation.

As people differ in such matters, so also do societies. Virtually all developed countries spend a larger percentage of government resources for social programs than the United States, although most other countries' per capita spending levels are lower. For example, in 1946 Great Britain established a nationalized health care system, with access to care for all citizens. *In terms of percentage of gross national product, Great Britain currently spends only about half as much per capita on health care as the United States, yet British citizens, by most indicators, are at least as healthy as Americans.*

The British system is organized on the basis of local areas, each with a predetermined annual budget. Resources are limited within this closed system: funds not spent on one health-related product are spent on another such product. In contrast, the United States has an open system. Since dollars in this system are not limited by budgets in the same way as in Great Britain, what is not spent on one health-related product may or may not be spent on another. Given a similar set of public needs, the United States and Great Britain have made different allocation decisions.

Resources are not infinitely available in any delivery system, and thus potentially beneficial care must sometimes be denied. Theoretically, denial occurs when society (or a provider acting on its behalf) judges the marginal cost of a service to be more than its marginal benefit; the service is therefore withheld. Although the service may well be one that would benefit the individual, society may determine that the resources involved could be better spent elsewhere.

The British make explicit tradeoffs between health and other goods, particularly as they relate to resource-intensive services; and for the most part this decision process treats all people in the system on an equal basis. The U.S. health care system has a different, more implicit, set of priorities, but resources are rationed nonetheless; some receive services, others do not. To a large degree these decisions depend on characteristics of the individual patient (insurance status, socioeconomic status) or the provider (geographic location, reimbursement incentives). As a result,

"Saying no to beneficial treatments or procedures in the United States is morally hard, because providers cannot appeal to the justice of their denial. In ideally just arrangements, and even in the British system, rationing beneficial care is nevertheless fair to all patients in general. Cost-containment measures in our system carry with them no such justification" (Daniels 1986, p. 1383).

To be sure, U.S. physicians and other practitioners, possessing the technical knowledge that they do, can make valuable contributions to national policy formulations. What they cannot ethically do is participate in any formal rationing process involving individual patients, since doing so would weaken the physician's responsibility as the patient's agent. In short, the problem of allocating the nation's health care resources requires the practitioner to wear more than one hat, and to decide when and where it is appropriate to wear each. This is no easy decision, but there is no escaping it. Today's physician has a duty to consider the balance between the needs of the individual and those of society.

Tomorrow's Practitioner: Tradesman or Professional?

Since 1975, when physicians' exemption from the antitrust laws was lifted, the law has treated medicine as a trade rather than a profession. Ten years later it was suggested that the public is coming to share this perspective (King 1985). The distinction is more than a matter of semantics: it will directly affect the ethical responsibilities and societal role of future physicians. Throughout this century, physicians have been among the most respected members of our society, and deservedly so. But to retain that respect, they must show very clearly that they are more than tradesmen.

Today's health care providers are living through a period of accelerated change. Many issues are on the table, involving not only the health care industry but the legal and political systems. As the organization and financing of U.S. health care are reshaped, the ability to accept change and adapt to new conditions will be necessary. The role practitioners play in resolving these issues will go a long way toward determining the future of the medical profession in the new medical marketplace.

We believe that practitioners should assume direct responsibility for some of today's issues. They should forthrightly address such matters as the role of ethics and costs in individual clinical decisions and such complex societal problems as charity care and medical malpractice. They should form considered views on the optimum allocation of health care resources and take the necessary steps to get those views heard by those who make the decisions, whether by writing articles for journals, lecturing, serving as consultants, or serving on appropriate committees or boards. And they should educate their patients and the public on the important effects that lifestyle has on health.

We are also in favor of political activity, both individual and collective, assuming that it maximizes the role of medical expertise and does not give the appearance of being totally self-serving. A group of physicians representing "organized medicine" and presenting a unified front before legislators on a particular issue not only serves as an appropriate interface between the political system, society, and the medical profession, but can get things done that the ordinary political process might never get around to.

Perhaps the most important way of ensuring that physicians continue to be accorded professional status is for the profession to establish sensible and believable mechanisms for disciplining delinquent members, for licensing, for continuing education, and for reviewing and assuring the quality of care. Such measures are a must if payers, patients, and policymakers are to be convinced that today's physicians take their mission seriously and are willing to acknowledge accountability for their behavior.

Values cherished by all parties are at stake, and what should be a cooperative enterprise sometimes looks more like a battle. A new equilibrium has yet to be reached, and even its general outlines are not yet as clear as one might wish. Change is everywhere. But some important things will not change. In the words of Carola Eisenberg of the Harvard Medical School (1986, p. 1114), *"The satisfaction of being able to relieve pain and restore function, the intellectual challenge of solving clinical problems, and the variety of human issues we confront in daily clinical practice will remain the essence of doctoring, whatever the changes in the organizational and economic structure of medicine."*

ACRONYMS, ABBREVIATIONS, AND TERMS

AARP. American Association of Retired Persons.

access to care. A person's ability to obtain health care when needed. To obtain access, the provider must be available, affordable, appropriate, and acceptable to the patient.

ADS. Alternative delivery system: a generic term for any "new" health provider organization or system seen as an alternative to traditional health insurance plans. ADSs usually involve a significant degree of vertical integration and prearranged contracts between insurers and providers. HMOs and PPOs are ADSs. (See also *managed care* and *CMP.*)

AHA. American Hospital Association.

AMA. American Medical Association.

assignment. A provider who accepts assignment submits a bill directly to the insurer and accepts the company's reimbursement as payment in full for the service. The patient may or may not still be responsible for any cost-sharing provisions, depending on the insurance plan. A provider who accepts assignment will not "balance-bill." (See also *balance billing, Participating Physician,* and p. 71.)

ATRA. American Tort Reform Association.

AVGs. Ambulatory Visit Groups: a potential per-case reimbursement method for outpatient care. (See p. 94.)

balance-billing. Direct billing of an insured patient by a provider. The patient is then personally responsible for payment of any charge exceeding the insurer's allowed reimbursement. (See also *assignment* and p. 72.)

capitation. A system of financing in which a provider is paid a per capita fee for each consumer, which is negotiated before the consumer receives any care. (See Chapter 6.)

case manager. A patient's representative hired by an insurer or corporate employer who coordinates the care process, especially as it relates to high-cost or long-term care. (See alternative definition under *gatekeeper.*)

CBA. Cost-benefit analysis: an evaluation method in which monetary values are assigned to both the inputs and outcomes of a health care technology or program. CBA is used to assist in decisions regarding the allocation of resources among alternative technologies or programs.

CEA. Cost-effectiveness analysis: an evaluation method in which the inputs of a health care technology or program are measured in monetary units but outcomes are measured in nonmonetary units (such as years of life saved or morbidity avoided). CEA is used by decision makers to compare programs or treatments with similar effects.

CMP. Competitive Medical Plan: HCFA's term for HMOs that are not federally qualified. They provide service to Medicare beneficiaries on a "risk-sharing" capitated payment basis. The term CMP is sometimes also used interchangeably with ADS. (See also p. 66.)

CON. Certificate-of-Need program: a program coordinated by state planning agencies that requires health care facilities to obtain approval before they make major investments in equipment or services. (See also p. 81.)

cost-plus reimbursement. An FFS payment system where the provider (usually a hospital) is retrospectively paid its actual costs for providing a service, plus a preset percentage as "mark-up." (See also p. 69.)

cost-sharing. An insurance arrangement by which insured consumers are required to pay a portion of their medical bills out of pocket. Deductibles, co-payments, and co-insurance are all types of cost-sharing. (See also Chapter 6.)

CPR. Customary-Prevailing-Reasonable: a method used by Medicare for determining the allowable amount to be paid a provider under FFS payment. (See also *UCR*; p. 70; and Table 7, p. 71.)

CPT. Current Procedural Terminology: a taxonomy of procedure codes developed by the AMA, primarily for purposes of billing.

CRVS. California Relative Value Scale: a scale, developed by the California Medical Association, in which each procedure is assigned a weight for use in determining its "relative value" compared to other procedures. (See also *RVS; fee schedule;* and p. 75.)

CT. Computerized tomography (scanner).

deductible. A type of insurance cost-sharing in which a beneficiary pays a predetermined dollar amount out-of-pocket for medical services before any insurance benefits are reimbursed.

demand creation. The ability of medical care providers to initiate demand for their services, such as by scheduling return office visits.

When a consumer does not truly require the service, initiation of the service is considered inducement. (See also p. 50.)

DO. Doctor of Osteopathic Medicine.

DRGs. Diagnosis Related Groups: a set of categories, based on patient diagnosis, procedures, and age, assigned for purposes of PPS hospital reimbursement (primarily under Medicare). (See also p. 88.)

EPO. Exclusive Provider Organization: a type of PPO in which patients are required to use providers within the PPO.

FEC. Freestanding emergency-care center: a non-hospital-based ambulatory care facility providing extended-hour emergency services. Similar types of facilities providing ambulatory care to nonemergency patients have been termed urgent-care (or urgi-care) centers and convenience-care centers. (See also p. 103.)

fee schedule. A system, often based on an RVS, whereby third-party payers reimburse a predetermined amount for a given service, regardless of the provider-designated fee. (See also *RVS* and p. 73.)

FFS. Fee-for-service reimbursement: an arrangement in which a provider charges a fee for each separate service; payment is made after the service is provided. (See also Chapter 7.)

for-profit health care. Health care provided by a corporation whose surplus income is paid to those who own or have invested in the corporation. (See also *nonprofit health care*.)

gatekeeper. A primary care physician who manages the case of an individual patient by coordinating all services. In some health plans, no specialist or hospital care will be reimbursed without the gatekeeper's prior approval. (See also *case manager*.)

GMENAC. Graduate Medical Education National Advisory Committee: a blue-ribbon government panel that studied, among other issues, the adequacy of the U.S. health care manpower supply in the 1980s. (See also p. 44.)

GNP. Gross national product.

HCFA. U.S. Health Care Financing Administration: the agency responsible for Medicare and the federal involvement in Medicaid. Part of the U.S. Department of Health and Human Services. (See also *Medicare, Medicaid*.)

health insurance. Insurance offering consumer protection against medical expenses in return for a fixed, predetermined premium. Usually covers hospital and professional fees. Blue Cross/Blue Shield is the major "nonprofit" private insurer in the U.S. The "commercials" are the private for-profit health insurers. (See also Chapter 6.)

HIAA. Health Insurance Association of America.

HMO. Health maintenance organization: a prepaid delivery system in which the organization (and usually its primary care physicians) assume financial risk for the care provided to enrolled members. The HMO is legally committed to provide care to its enrollees, and members must obtain care from within the system if it is to be reimbursed. (See also Chapters 6, 7, and 8.)

horizontal integration. An arrangement by which a corporation (either for-profit or nonprofit) operates or coordinates a number of health care facilities providing the same level of service, e.g., a chain of hospitals. (See also *vertical integration.*)

HSAs. Health Systems Agencies: regional planning bodies created in the 1970s to assess local needs for medical care resources.

ICD-9. International Classification of Diseases, 9th revision: a taxonomy of approximately 10,000 diagnoses and 5,000 procedure codes. The DRG system is based on these codes.

IPA. Independent (or Individual) Practice Association: a type of HMO in which independent physicians contract with the HMO corporation to provide care to its enrolled members. (See also *HMO.*)

IV. Intravenous.

LOS. Length of stay (in-hospital).

MAAC. Maximum allowable annual charge: a mandated cap placed on the charge submitted to Medicare by a nonparticipating physician. (See *CPR* and p. 71.)

managed care. A term often used generically for all types of ADSs (e.g., HMOs and PPOs), implying that they "manage" the care received by consumers; the contrast is with traditional FFS care, which is unmanaged. The term is also used to describe a range of utilization controls that are applied to "manage" the practices of physicians and other providers, regardless of whether or not they are in an ADS. (See also *MIP* and *ADS.*)

MD-DRGs. Physician DRGs: a potential reimbursement method in which the admitting physician receives a DRG-based flat fee to provide all hospital-based care for an illness episode. (See also p. 92.)

Medicaid. A joint federal-state health insurance program (or more correctly entitlement program) for poor Americans, administered mainly by state governments. (See also pp. 38 and 56.)

Medicare. A national health insurance program for Americans over 65 and the disabled. The program is administered by HCFA. Part A of the program covers hospital expenses; Part B covers physicians and other professional services. (See also pp. 40 and 56.)

MEI. Medicare Economic Index: an HCFA formula limiting yearly increases in Medicare Part B reimbursement, based on practice cost increases and general wage levels. (See also pp. 71 and 85.)

MeSH. Medical Staff and Hospital: a "joint venture" in which a hospital and its private-practice medical staff form a legal corporation, which may then contract to care for enrollees in an HMO or a PPO, or itself becomes an HMO or a PPO.

MIP. Managed Indemnity Plan: a type of ADS in which a health insurance company, often representing a self-insured employer, mandates standards of practice for providers who wish to be reimbursed via FFS for care provided to enrollees. MIPs rely on a range of utilization controls including prehospital certification, second-opinion surgery, and case managers. (See also *managed care* and p. 100.)

national health insurance. A program in which government provides (or certifies) health insurance for all citizens; alternatively, the program may employ providers directly. Such a system is in place in Canada, Great Britain, and virtually all other developed countries.

NIH. National Institutes of Health.

nonprofit health care. Health care provided by an organization (usually a corporation) whose surplus income is reinvested in the organization itself. (See also *for-profit* health care.)

OEO. Office of Economic Opportunity: a government unit developed during the 1960s to lead the war on poverty. This office was responsible for a program of "Neighborhood Health Centers." (See also p. 29.)

Participating Physician. A provider who agrees to accept assignment from Medicare (or another insurer) for individual patients or all beneficiaries treated during a specified time period. (See also *assignment* and p. 71.)

per-case payment. A reimbursement method in which the provider receives a flat fee to provide all care for a given patient "case" (i.e., illness episode). The payment amount is usually prenegotiated and usually not dependent on the type or amount of services provided. The DRG-based PPS system is a per-case payment system.

PPGP. Prepaid group practice: a type of HMO in which a large group (or groups) of physicians provide medical services to enrollees of the plan. The group usually receives payment on a capitated basis. If the group is incorporated separately from the HMO, it is considered a group-model HMO. If the physicians practice in a group primarily salaried by the HMO, it is considered a staff-model HMO. (See also *HMO* and p. 27.)

PPO. Preferred provider organization: an ADS that acts as a broker between the purchaser and the provider of care. Providers usually receive payment on a discounted FFS basis. Enrollees are given incentives (e.g., no co-insurance) to use providers within the PPO, but they may seek covered services from outside the PPO system.

PPS. Prospective Payment System: a hospital reimbursement system for Medicare's Part A, in which the provider is reimbursed a prospectively determined, fixed amount per patient admission regardless of the quantity of services received by that patient. (See also *DRG, per-case payment*, and p. 88.)

PRO. Peer Review Organization: a public-sector-funded utilization review (UR) program, composed of independent contracting physician groups in each state. PROs are charged with monitoring the cost and quality of care received by Medicare beneficiaries. To date PROs review hospital care and Medicare-participating HMOs. Professional Standards Review Organizations (PSROs) were the predecessors of PROs. (See p. 83.)

QA. Quality assurance (program): a program implemented in many hospitals (and other facilities) to ensure a high quality of care. Many QA programs are also responsible for UR. (See also *UR.*)

RAP. Radiology, Anesthesiology, Pathology: an acronym used largely in reimbursement negotiations with HCFA.

risk-sharing. A payment arrangement in which a provider accepts at least some risk of decreased reimbursement if his or her performance is inefficient. Capitation payment systems involve risk-sharing, as do systems where a certain percentage of the provider's FFS payments (e.g., 20 percent) are "held back" in escrow, pending an evaluation—usually annual—of the financial performance of the physician or the plan. In general, all HMOs incorporate risk-sharing.

RUGs. Resource Utilization Groups: a per-case reimbursement method for nursing home care. (See also p. 94.)

RVS. Relative Value Scale: a system for weighting the value of different medical services. An RVS is often used to develop a fee schedule. (See also *CRVS, fee schedule*, and p. 74.)

RVU. Relative Value Unit: the weighting unit in an RVS system.

self-insurance. An arrangement in which an employer acts as "health insurer" by paying employees' medical expenses directly rather than by paying their insurance premiums. Most self-insured employers contract out the administration of such plans. Also some purchase "minimal insurance" to cover very expensive events (e.g., an employee's use of over $50,000 worth of services).

S/HMO. Social Health Maintenance Organization: a new type of HMO developed on a demonstration basis with HCFA funding, intended to expand HMO services to provide social support and long-term care to elderly and disabled Medicare enrollees.

small-area variation. Variation in the medical services provided in different geographic locales. Such variation is identified by epidemiological comparisons of the practice patterns of populations of clinicians in different areas. (See also p. 130.)

TA. Technology assessment: the evaluation of a new medical technique or technology, usually through comparison of patient outcomes with those obtained by using existing technologies. TA also involves an assessment of resource inputs and the value of outputs. (See also *CBA* and *CEA*.)

third-party payers. Those who reimburse providers for health care services, as distinguished from the patient and the provider (the first two parties). In the United States the major third parties are the U.S. government (which is responsible for Medicare and Medicaid), the nonprofit Blue Cross/Blue Shield plans, and the commercial insurers. Through their involvement in self-insured plans, corporations can also be considered an important third party.

UCR. Usual-Customary-Reasonable: a method used by insurers for determining amounts paid under FFS reimbursement. (See also *CPR*; p. 70; and Table 7, p. 71.)

uncompensated care. Medical services provided to a patient for which no reimbursement is received. Uncompensated care is provided mainly to uninsured Americans.

UR. Utilization review: a case-by-case evaluation of the use of clinical resources in which actual practices are compared to predetermined criteria. (See also *QA* and p. 82.)

VA. Veterans Administration.

vertical integration. An arrangement by which a corporation (either for-profit or nonprofit) operates or coordinates a group of facilities that collectively offer many levels of health care services. A vertically integrated organization usually provides or arranges for the delivery of primary care, specialized ambulatory care, hospital care, and long-term care. An HMO can be viewed as a type of vertically integrated organization. (See also *horizontal integration*.)

REFERENCES/BIBLIOGRAPHY

Chapter 2

Ackernecht, Erwin. 1982. *A Short History of Medicine*, rev. ed. Baltimore: Johns Hopkins University Press.

"An Overcrowded Profession—the Cause and the Remedy." 1901. *JAMA* 37, 12: 775–776.

Anderson, Odin. 1985. *Health Services in the United States: A Growth Enterprise since 1875*. Ann Arbor, Mich.: Health Administration Press.

Bergman, Norman. 1985. "Forerunners of Modern Anesthesiology: Dwarfs and Giants." *The Pharos*, Fall, pp. 8–12.

Berliner, Howard. 1975. "A Larger Perspective on the Flexner Report." *International Journal of Health Services* 5, 4: 573–592.

Bordley, James, and A. McGehee Harvey. 1976. *Two Centuries of American Medicine: 1776–1976*. Philadelphia: W. B. Saunders.

Buhler-Wilkerson, Karen. 1985. "Public Health Nursing: In Sickness or in Health?" *AmJPubHealth* 75, 10: 1155–1161.

Califano, Joseph. 1986. "A Corporage Rx for America: Managing Runaway Health Costs." *Issues in Science and Technology*, Spring, pp. 81–90.

Commission on Hospital Care. 1947. *Hospital Care in the United States*. New York: Commonwealth Fund.

Committee on the Costs of Medical Care. 1932. *Medical Care for the American People—Final Report*. Chicago: University of Chicago Press.

Corning, Peter. 1969. *The Evolution of Medicare . . . From Idea to Law*. Social Security Administration, Office of Research and Statistics, Research Report 29. Washington, D.C.: GPO.

Editors of *Fortune*. 1970. *Our Ailing Medical System: It's Time to Operate*. New York: Harper and Row.

Evans, Bergan. 1978. *Dictionary of Quotations*. New York: Avenel Books.

Fein, Rashi. 1962. *The Doctor Shortage: An Economic Diagnosis*. Washington, D.C.: Brookings Institution.

Fleming, Donald. 1954. *William H. Welch and the Rise of Modern Medicine*. Boston: Little, Brown.

Freymann, John. 1974. *The American Health Care System: Its Genesis and Trajectory*. New York: Medcom Press.

Fuchs, Victor. 1974. *Who Shall Live? Health, Economics, and Social Choice*. New York: Basic Books.

Garrison, Fielding. 1929. *An Introduction to the History of Medicine*. Philadelphia: W. B. Saunders.

Gillick, Muriel. 1985. "Common-Sense Models of Health and Disease." *NEnglJMed* 313, 11: 700–703.

Gornick, Marion, J. Greenberg, P. Eggers, and A. Dobson. 1985. "Twenty Years of Medicare and Medicaid: Covered Populations, Use of Benefits, and Program Expenditures." *Health Care Financing Review*, Annual Supplement, pp. 13–62.

Hatfield, Charles. 1920. "Relative Functions of Health Agencies: II. Viewpoint of the Non-Official Agency." *AmJPubHealth* 10, 12: 948–952.

Hearings Before the Committee on Education and Labor. 1945. United States Senate. Bill S.191. February and March 1945. Washington, D.C.: GPO.

Hirshfield, Daniel. 1970. *The Lost Reform: The Campaign for Compulsory Health Insurance in the United States from 1932 to 1943.* Cambridge, Mass.: Harvard University Press.

Howell, Joel. 1986. "Early Use of X-ray Machines and Electrocardiographs at the Pennsylvania Hospital: 1897 Through 1927." *JAMA* 255, 17: 2320–2323.

King, Lester. 1984. "The Flexner Report of 1910." *JAMA* 251, 8: 1079–1086.

Kingsdale, Jon. 1981. *The Growth of Hospitals: An Economic History in Baltimore*, vol. 1. Ann Arbor, Mich.: University Microfilms International.

Knowles, John, ed. 1977. *Doing Better and Feeling Worse: Health in the United States.* New York: W. W. Norton.

Kuhn, Thomas. 1962. *The Structure of Scientific Revolutions.* Chicago: University of Chicago Press.

Lewis, Irving, and Cecil Sheps. 1983. *The Sick Citadel.* Cambridge, Mass.: Oelgeschlager, Gunn and Hain.

Reed, Louis. 1933. *The Ability to Pay for Medical Care.* Publication of the Committee on the Costs of Medical Care. Chicago: University of Chicago Press.

Reiser, Stanley. 1984. "The Machine at the Bedside: Technological Transformations of Practices and Values." In *Machine at the Bedside*, edited by Stanley Reiser and Michael Anbar. New York: Cambridge University Press.

Ricardo-Campbell, Rita. 1982. *The Economics and Politics of Health.* Chapel Hill: University of North Carolina Press.

Roemer, Milton. 1985. "I. S. Falk, the Committee on the Costs of Medical Care, and the Drive for National Health Insurance." *AmJPubHealth* 75, 8: 841–848.

Roemer, Milton. 1986. *An Introduction to the U.S. Health Care System.* New York: Springer Publishing.

Rosen, George. 1958. *A History of Public Health.* New York: MD Publications.

Sardell, Alice. 1983. "Neighborhood Health Centers and Community-Based Care: Federal Policy from 1965 to 1982." *Journal of Public Health Policy* 4, 4: 484–503.

Shorter, Edward. 1985. *Bedside Manners.* New York: Simon and Schuster.

Shryock, Richard. 1962. *Medicine and Society in America: 1660–1860.* Ithaca, N.Y.: Great Seal Book.

Spingarn, Natalie. 1976. *Heartbeat: The Politics of Health Research.* Washington, D.C.: Robert B. Luce.

Starr, Paul. 1982. *The Social Transformation of American Medicine.* New York: Basic Books.

Tarlov, Alvin. 1983. "The Increasing Supply of Physicians, the Changing Structure of the Health-Services System, and the Future Practice of Medicine." *NEnglJMed* 308, 20: 1235–1244.

Thomas, Lewis. 1983. *The Youngest Science: Notes of a Medicine-Watcher.* New York: Viking Press.

United States Department of Health and Human Services. 1982. *Health Care Financing Program Statistics: The Medicare and Medicaid Data Book, 1981.* HHS Publication. HCFA Pub. No. 03128.

United States General Accounting Office. 1985. *Constraining National Health Care Expenditures: Achieving Quality Care at an Affordable Cost.* Pub. GAO/HRD-85-105.

Walsh, Diana, and Richard Egdahl. 1977. *Payer, Provider, Consumer: Industry Confronts Health Care Costs.* New York: Springer-Verlag.

Williams, Greer. 1971. *Kaiser-Permanente Health Plan: Why It Works.* Oakland, Calif.: Kaiser Foundation.

Young, Hugh. 1910. "After Fifteen Years: A Glance at Recent Progress in Medicine and Surgery." In *History of Surgery.* Charlottesville, Va.: Michie Company.

Ziporyn, Terra. 1985. "The Food and Drug Administration: How 'Those Regulations' Came to Be." *JAMA* 254, 15: 2037–2046.

Chapter 3

"AMA Insights." 1985. *JAMA* 254, 6: 746.

Anderson, Odin. 1985. *Health Services in the United States: A Growth Enterprise since 1875.* Ann Arbor, Mich.: Health Administration Press.

Blendon, Robert, and David Rogers. 1983. "Cutting Medical Care Costs: *Primum Non Nocere.*" *JAMA* 250, 14: 1880–1885.

Blumenthal, David. 1986. "Prescriptions for America's Health Care System." *Washington Post Book World,* 13 April, pp. 1–2.

Califano, Joseph. 1986. "A Corporate Rx for America: Managing Runaway Health Costs." *Issues in Science and Technology,* Spring, pp. 81–90.

Employee Benefit Research Institute. 1986. "Features of Employer Health Plans: Cost Containment, Plan Funding and Coverage Continuation." Washington, D.C.

Freedman, Steven, 1985. "Megacorporate Health Care: A Choice for the Future." *NEnglJMed* 312, 9: 579–582.

Fry, J., and J. Hasler. 1986. *Primary Health Care 2000.* Edinburgh: Churchill Livingstone.

HCFA, Division of National Cost Estimates. 1987. "National Health Expenditures, 1986–2000." *Health Care Financing Review,* 8, 4: 1–36.

Health Insurance Association of America. 1987. *1986–1987 Source Book of Health Insurance Data.* Washington, D.C.

Iglehart, John. 1985. "The Veterans Administration Medical Care System Faces an Uncertain Future." *NEnglJMed* 313, 18: 1168–1172.

Illich, Ivan. 1976. *Medical Nemesis: The Expropriation of Health.* New York: Random House.

Jonas, Steven. 1986. *Health Care Delivery in the United States,* 3rd ed. New York: Springer Publishing.

Rublee, Dale. 1985. "Self-Funded Health Benefit Plans: Trends, Legal Environment, and Policy Issues." *JAMA* 255, 6: 787–789.

Sardell, Alice. 1983. "Neighborhood Health Centers and Community-Based Care: Federal Policy from 1965 to 1982." *Journal of Public Health Policy* 4, 4: 484–503.

Schieber, G., and J. P. Poullier. 1986. "International Health Care Spending." *Health Affairs* 5, 3: 111–122.

Schramm, Carl. 1983. "The Teaching Hospital and the Future Role of State Government." *NEnglJMed* 308, 1: 41–45.

Sorkin, Alan, 1986. *Health Care and the Changing Economic Environment.* Lexington, Mass.: D. C. Heath and Company.

Starr, Paul. 1982. *The Social Transformation of American Medicine.* New York: Basic Books.

Steinwachs, Donald, Jonathan Weiner, Sam Shapiro, *et al.* 1986. "A Comparison of the Requirements for Primary Care Physicians in HMOs with Projections Made by the Graduate Education National Advisory Committee." *NEnglJMed* 314, 4: 217–222.

"A Survey of Public Opinion Trends Affecting Government and the Economy." 1982. *Opinion Outlook* 2, no. 3 (12 February).

Thurow, Lester. 1984. "Learning to Say No." *NEnglJMed* 311, 24: 1569–1572.

USDHHS. 1985. *Health. United States. 1985.* USDHHS (PHS) 86–1232. Washington, D.C.: GPO.

USDHHS, Health Resources Administration, Office of Graduate Medical Education. 1980. *Report of the Graduate Medical Education National Advisory Committee to the Secretary, Department of Health and Human Services,* vols. 1–8. Pub. by the U.S. Department of HHS, Public Health Service, Health Resources Administration, Office of Graduate Medical Education. Washington, D.C.

U.S. General Accounting Office. 1985. *Constraining National Health Care Expenditures: Achieving Quality Care at an Affordable Cost.* Pub. GAO/HRD-85-105.

Waldo, Daniel, Katharine Levit, and Helen Lazenby. 1986. "National Health Expenditures, 1985." *Health Care Financing Review* 8, 1: 1–21.

Walsh, Diana, and Richard Egdahl. 1977. *Payer, Provider, Consumer: Industry Confronts Health Care Costs.* New York: Springer-Verlag.

Chapter 4

Aaron, Henry, and William Schwartz. 1984. *The Painful Prescription.* Washington, D.C.: Brookings Institution.

Bailey, Richard. 1977. "An Economist's View of the Health Services Industry." In *Economics in Health Care,* edited by Lewis Weeks and Howard Berman, pp. 23–37. Germantown, Md.: Aspen Publication.

Commission on Hospital Care. 1947. *Hospital Care in the U.S.* New York: Commonwealth Fund.

Cowan, Belita. 1987. *Health Care Shoppers Guide: 59 Ways to Save Money.* Published by the Consumer Protection Division of the Maryland Attorney General's Office. Baltimore.

Eisenberg, John. 1986. *Doctors' Decisions and the Cost of Medical Care.* Ann Arbor, Mich.: Health Administration Press.

Enthoven, Alain. 1978a. "Consumer-Choice Health Plan: Inflation and Inequity in Health Care Today: Alternatives for Cost Control and an Analysis of Proposals for National Health Insurance." *NEnglJMed* 298, 12: 650–658.

Enthoven, Alain. 1978b. "Consumer-Choice Health Plan: A National-Health-

Insurance Proposal Based on Regulated Competition in the Private Sector." *NEnglJMed* 298, 13: 709–720.

Feldstein, Paul, 1983. *Health Care Economics*, 2nd ed. New York: John Wiley and Sons.

Gabel, Jon, and Michael Redisch. 1979. "Alternative Physician Payment Methods: Incentives, Efficiency, and National Health Insurance." *Milbank Memorial Fund Quarterly* 57, 1: 38–59.

Ginzberg, Eli. 1983a. "The Grand Illusion of Competition in Health Care." *JAMA* 249, 14: 1857–1859.

Ginzberg, Eli. 1983b. "Cost Containment—Imaginary and Real." *NEnglJMed* 308, 20: 1220–1224.

Hsiao, William, and William Stason. 1979. "Toward Developing a Relative Value Scale for Medical and Surgical Services." *Health Care Financing Review* 1, 2: 23–37.

Joseph, Hyman. 1977. "Empirical Research on the Demand for Health Care." In *Economics in Health Care*, edited by Lewis Weeks and Howard Berman, pp. 65–75. Germantown, Md.: Aspen Publication.

"Medicare: Paying the Physician—History, Issues, and Options." 1984. An information paper prepared for use by The Special Committee on Aging of the United States Senate. Washington, D.C.: GPO.

National Center for Health Statistics. 1985. *Health. United States. 1985.* DHHS Pub. No. (PHS) 86–1323. Public Health Service. Washington, D.C.: GPO.

Pear, Robert. 1987. "38.5% Rise Asked in 1988 Premiums of Medicare Users." *New York Times*, September 15, p. 1.

Reinhardt, Uwe. 1980. *On the Future of the American Economy and Its Impact on the Health Care Sector.* Chicago: University of Chicago Press.

Relman, Arnold. 1983. "The Future of Medical Practice." *Health Affairs* 2, 2: 5–19.

Relman, Arnold. 1985. "Antitrust Law and the Physician Entrepreneur." *NEnglJMed* 313, 14: 884–885.

Rosenblum, Robert. 1985. "Medicare Revisited: A Look Through the Past to the Future." *Journal of Health Politics, Policy and Law* 9, 4: 669–681.

Somers, Anne. 1987. "Insurance for Long-Term Care: Some Definitions, Problems, and Guidelines for Action." *NEnglJMed* 317, 1: 23–29.

Sorkin, Alan. 1975. *Health Economics: An Introduction.* Lexington, Mass.: D. C. Heath and Company.

U.S. General Accounting Office. 1985. *Constraining National Health Care Expenditures: Achieving Quality Care at an Affordable Cost.* Pub. GAO/HRD-85-105.

Wilensky, Gail, and Louis Rossiter. 1983. "The Relative Importance of Physician-Induced Demand in the Demand for Medical Care." *Milbank Memorial Fund Quarterly* 61, 2: 252–277.

Chapter 5

Aiken, Linda, and Karl Bays. 1984. "The Medicare Debate—Round One." *NEnglJMed* 311, 18: 1196–1200.

AMA. 1986. "Socioeconomic Characteristics of Medical Practice 1986." Chicago: AMA.

Anderson, Gerard, and James Studnicki. 1985. "Insurers Competing with Providers." *Hospitals* 59, 23: 64–66.

Arnett, Ross, and Gordon Tranell. 1984. "Private Health Insurance: New Measures of a Complex and Changing Industry." *Health Care Financing Review* 6, 1: 31–42.

Blumenthal, David, Mark Schlesinger, Pamela Drumheller, and the Harvard Medicare Project. 1986. "The Future of Medicare." *NEnglJMed* 314, 11: 722–728.

Brook, Robert, John Ware, William Rogers, *et al.* 1983. "Does Free Care Improve Adults' Health?: Results from a Randomized Controlled Trial." *NEnglJMed* 209, 23: 1426–1434.

Davis, Karen, and Diane Rowland. 1986. *Medicare Policy: New Directions for Health and Long-Term Care.* Baltimore: Johns Hopkins University Press.

Ellwood, Deborah. 1986. "Medicare Risk Contracting: Promises and Problems." *Health Affairs* 5, 1: 183–189.

Enthoven, Alain. 1984. "A New Proposal to Reform the Tax Treatment of Health Insurance." *Health Affairs* 3, 1: 21–39.

Gabel, Jon, and Dan Ermann. 1985. "Preferred Provider Organizations: Performance, Problems, and Promise." *Health Affairs* 4, 1: 24–40.

Ginsburg, Paul, and Glenn Hackbarth. 1986. "Alternative Delivery Systems and Medicare." *Health Affairs* 5, 1: 6–22.

Ginzberg, Eli. 1985. "The Restructuring of U.S. Health Care." *Inquiry* 22, 3: 272–281.

Harris, Seymour. 1975. *The Economics of Health Care: Financing and Delivery.* Berkeley, Calif.: McCutcheon Publishing Corporation.

HCFA. 1986. *The Medicare and Medicaid Data Book 1984.* HCFA Publication No. 03210. Baltimore.

HCFA. 1987. "National Health Expenditures." *Health Care Financing Review* 8, 4: 1–22.

Health Insurance Association of America. 1985. *Survey of Group Health Insurance Programs.* Washington, D.C.

Iglehart, John. 1985. "The Veterans Administration Medical Care System and the Private Sector." *NEnglJMed* 313, 24: 1552–1556.

Jacobs, Phil. 1980. *The Economics of Health and Medical Care.* Baltimore: University Park Press.

Juba, David. 1985. "Medicare Part B: A Time for Reform." *Business and Health,* November, pp. 5–8.

Kleinfield, N. R. 1986. "When the Boss Becomes Your Doctor." *New York Times,* January 5, pp. F1, F3.

Luft, Harold. 1978. "How Do Health-Maintenance Organizations Achieve Their 'Savings'?: Rhetoric and Evidence." *NEnglJMed* 298, 24: 1336–1343.

Marquis, Susan, and Kathleen Lohr. 1984. "Medicare and Medicaid: Past, Present, and Future." A Rand Corporation report prepared for the Department of Health and Human Services. Santa Monica, Calif.

Moore, Stephen, Diane Martin, and William Richardson. 1983. "Does the Primary-Care Gatekeeper Control the Costs of Health Care?: Lessons from the SAFECO Experience." *NEnglJMed* 309, 22: 1400–1404.

Newhouse, Joseph. 1978. "Insurance Benefits, Out-Of-Pocket Payments, and the Demand for Medical Care." *Health and Medical Care Services Review* 1, 4: 1–15.

Newhouse, Joseph, Willard Manning, Carl Morris, *et al.* 1981. "Some Interim Results from a Controlled Trial of Cost Sharing in Health Insurance." *NEnglJMed* 305, 25: 1501–1507.

Reiser, Stanley, and Michael Anbar, eds. 1984. *Machine at the Bedside.* New York: Cambridge University Press.

Saward, Ernest, and E. K. Gallagher. 1983. "Reflections on Change in Medical Practice: The Current Trend to Large-Scale Medical Organizations." *JAMA* 250, 20: 2820–2825.

Siu, Albert, Frank Sonnenberg, Willard Manning, *et al.* 1986. "Inappropriate Use of Hospitals in a Randomized Trial of Health Insurance Plans." *NEnglJMed* 315, 20: 1259–1266.

Sorkin, Alan. 1975. *Health Economics: An Introduction.* Lexington, Mass.: D. C. Heath and Company.

Sorkin, Alan. 1986. *Health Care and the Changing Economic Environment.* Lexington, Mass.: D. C. Heath and Company.

U.S. Congress, Office of Technology Assessment. 1986. *Payment for Physician Services: Strategies for Medicare.* OTA-H-294. Washington, D.C.: GPO.

USDHHS. 1987. *Health. U.S. 1986.* USDHHS (PHS) 87-1232. Washington, D.C.: GPO.

USDHHS, National Center for Health Services Research. 1982. "Prescribed Medicines, Users, and Expenditures." USDHHS (PHS) 82–3320.

USDHHS, National Center for Health Services Research. 1987. "A Summary of Expenditures and Sources of Payment for Personal Health Services." USDHHS (PHS) 87–3411.

Chapter 6

Aaron, Henry, and William Schwartz. 1984. *The Painful Prescription: Rationing Hospital Care.* Washington, D.C.: Brookings Institution.

American Medical Association. 1986. *Socioeconomic Characteristics of Medical Practice.* Chicago: AMA.

Burney, Ira, George Schieber, Martha Blaxall, and Jon Gabel. 1979. "Medicare and Medicaid Physician Payment Incentives." *Health Care Financing Review* 1, 1: 62–78.

Epstein, Arnold, Colin Begg, and Barbara McNeil. 1986. "The Use of Ambulatory Testing in Prepaid and Fee-for-Service Group Practices: Relation to Perceived Profitability." *NEnglJMed* 314, 17: 1089–1094.

Feldstein, Paul. 1983. *Health Care Economics*, 2nd ed. New York: John Wiley and Sons.

Gabel, Jon, and Michael Redisch. 1979. "Alternative Physician Payment Methods: Incentives, Efficiency, and National Health Insurance." *Milbank Memorial Fund Quarterly* 57, 1: 38–59.

Ginsburg, Paul, and Frank Sloan. 1984. "Hospital Cost Shifting." *NEnglJMed* 310, 14: 893–898.

Ginsburg, Paul, and Glenn Hackbarth. 1986. "Alternative Delivery Systems and Medicare." *Health Affairs* 5, 1: 6–22.

Harris, Seymour. 1975. *The Economics of Health Care.* Berkeley, Calif.: McCutcheon Publishing Corporation.

Health Policy Alternatives, Inc. 1986. "Physician Payment Reform under Medicare: Implications for Emergency Medicine." Report prepared for the American College of Emergency Physicians.

Holoweiko, Mark. 1986. "Non-Surgeons' Earnings: Which Specialties Are Hung Up?" *Medical Economics*, February 3, 206–225.

Hsiao, William, and William Stason. 1979. "Toward Developing a Relative Value Scale for Medical and Surgical Services." *Health Care Financing Review* 1, 2: 23–38.

Hsiao, William, Peter Braun, Edmund Becker, and Stephen Thomas. 1987. "The Resource-Based Relative Value Scale." *JAMA* 258, 6: 799–802.

Jencks, Stephen, and Allen Dobson. 1985. "Strategies for Reforming Medicare's Physician Payments." *NEnglJMed* 312, 23: 1492–1499.

Juba, David. 1985a. "Medicare Part B: A Time for Reform." *Business and Health*, November, pp. 5–8.

Juba, David, and Jack Hadley. 1985b. "Relative Value Scales for Physicians' Services." *Health Care Financing Review* 6, 4: 93–101.

Luft, Harold. 1981. *Health Maintenance Organizations: Dimensions of Performance*. New York: John Wiley and Sons.

Manning, Willard, Arleen Leibowitz, George Goldberg, William Rogers, and Joseph Newhouse. 1984. "Controlled Trial of the Effect of a Prepaid Group Practice on Use of Services." *NEnglJMed* 310, 23: 1505–1510.

O'Sullivan, Jennifer, and James Reuter. 1986. "Physician Reimbursement under Medicare." Report prepared for the Committee on Finance. Washington, D.C.: GPO.

Reinhardt, Uwe. 1985. "Future Trends in the Economics of Medical Practice and Care." *AmJCardiology* 56, 5: 50C–59C.

Relman, Arnold. 1985. "Cost Control, Doctors' Ethics, and Patient Care." *Issues in Science and Technology*, Winter, pp. 103–111.

Roe, Benson, 1981. "The UCR Boondoggle: A Death Knell for Private Practice?" *NEnglJMed* 305, 1: 41–45.

"Third-Party Funds Significant Part of Physicians' Revenues." 1985. *American Medical News*, October 4, p. 34.

U.S. Congress, Office of Technology Assessment. 1986. *Payment for Physician Services: Strategies for Medicare*. OTA-H-294. Washington, D.C.: GPO.

U.S. General Accounting Office. 1985. *Constraining National Health Care Expenditures: Achieving Quality Care at an Affordable Cost*. Pub. GAO/HRD-85-105. Washington, D.C.: GPO.

Chapter 7

Anderson, Gerard, and Earl Steinberg. 1984. "Hospital Readmissions in the Medicare Population." *NEnglJMed* 311, 21: 1249–1253.

Culler, Steven, and David Ehrenfried. 1986. "On the Feasibility and Usefulness of Physician DRGs." *Inquiry* 23, 1: 40–55.

Dans, Peter, Jonathan Weiner, and Sharon Otter. 1985. "Peer Review Organizations: Promises and Potential Pitfalls." *NEnglJMed* 311, 18: 1131–1137.

Davis, Karen, Gerard Anderson, Steven Renn, *et al.* 1985. "Is Cost Containment Working?" *Health Affairs* 4, 3: 81–94.

de Lissovoy, Greg, Thomas Rice, Dan Ermann, and Jon Gabel. 1986. "Preferred Provider Organizations: Today's Models and Tomorrow's Prospects." *Inquiry* 23, 1: 7–15.

Dolenc, Danielle, and Charles Dougherty. 1985. "DRGs: The Counterrevolution in Financing Health Care." *Hastings Center Report* 15, 3: 19–29.

Ellwood, Deborah. 1986. "Medicare Risk Contracting: Promises and Problems." *Health Affairs* 5, 1: 183–189.

Fielding, Jonathan. 1983. "Lessons from Health Care Regulation." *Annual Review of Public Health* 4: 91–130.

Frank, Richard, and Judith Lave. 1986. "Per Case Prospective Payment for Psychiatric Inpatients: An Assessment and Alternatives." *Journal of Health Politics, Policy and Law* 11, 1: 83–96.

Gabel, Jon, and Thomas Rice. 1985. "Reducing Public Expenditures for Physician Services: The Price of Paying Less." *Journal of Health Politics, Policy and Law* 9, 4: 595–609.

Gapen, Phyllis. 1985. "Empty Beds Are Major Problem in Maryland." *American Medical News*, December 27.

Ginsburg, Paul, and Glenn Hackbarth. 1986. "Alternative Delivery Systems and Medicare." *Health Affairs* 5, 1: 6–22.

Goldfield, Norbert, and Seth Goldsmith. 1987. *Alternative Delivery Systems*. Rockville, Md.: Aspen Publishers.

Guterman, Stuart, and Allen Dobson. 1986. "Impact of the Medicare Prospective Payment System for Hospitals." *Health Care Financing Review* 7, 3: 97–114.

HCFA. 1983. *The New ICD-9-CM Diagnosis Related Groups Classification Scheme*. Pub. 03167. Baltimore.

Iglehart, John. 1982. "The New Era of Prospective Payment for Hospitals." *NEnglJMed* 307, 20: 1288–1292.

Iglehart, John. 1986. "Early Experience with Prospective Payment of Hospitals." *NEnglJMed* 314, 22: 1460–1464.

Jencks, Stephen, and Allen Dobson. 1985. "Strategies for Reforming Medicare's Physician Payments." *NEnglJMed* 312, 23: 1492–1499.

Johns, Lucy. 1985. "Selective Contracting in California." *Health Affairs* 4, 3: 32–48.

Luft, Harold. 1985. "Competition and Regulation." *Medical Care* 23, 5: 383–399.

Maryland Hospital Association. 1986. *Research and Data Analysis*, no. 11.

Medicare: Paying the Physician—History, Issues, and Options. 1984. Paper prepared for use by The Special Committee on Aging, United States Senate. Washington, D.C.

Meiners, Mark, and Rosemary Coffey. 1985. "Hospital DRGs and the Need for Long-Term Care Services: An Empirical Analysis." *Health Services Research* 20, 3: 359–384.

Mitchell, Janet. 1985a. "Physician DRGs." *NEnglJMed* 313, 11: 670–675.

Mitchell, Janet. 1985b. "Physician DRGs: How Would They Work?" *Business and Health*, November, pp. 10–12.

Relman, Arnold. 1985. "Cost Control, Doctors' Ethics, and Patient Care." *Issues in Science and Technology*, Winter, pp. 103–111.

Roemer, Milton. 1981. *An Introduction to the U.S. Health Care System*. New York: Springer Publishing.

Roemer, Milton. 1985. "I. S. Falk, the Committee on the Costs of Medical Care, and the Drive for National Health Insurance." *AmJPubHealth* 75, 8: 841–848.

Schumacher, Dale, M. Jo Namerow, Barbara Parker, *et al.* 1986. "Prospective

Payment for Psychiatry—Feasibility and Impact." *NEnglJMed* 315, 21: 1331–1336.

Segal, Mark. 1985. "Diagnosis-Related Groups for Physician Reimbursement?" *JAMA* 254, 18: 2639–2640.

Simpson, James. 1985. "State Certificate-of-Need Programs: The Current Status." *AmJPubHealth* 75, 10: 1225–1229.

Sorkin, Alan. 1986. *Health Care and the Changing Economic Environment.* Lexington, Mass.: D. C. Heath and Company.

Steinwald, Bruce. 1986. "The Impact of New Reimbursement Schemes on Clinical Research in Hospitals: The Case of the Prospective Payment System." *Journal of General Internal Medicine* 1, supplement: S56-S59.

U.S. General Accounting Office. 1985. *Constraining National Health Care Expenditures: Achieving Quality Care at an Affordable Cost.* Pub. GAO/HRD-85-105. Washington, D.C.: GPO.

Walsh, Diana, and Richard Egdahl. 1977. *Payer, Provider, Consumer: Industry Confronts Health Care Costs.* New York: Springer-Verlag.

Young, David. 1985. "Physician Accountability for Health Care Costs." *Business and Health*, November, pp. 16–18.

Chapter 8

Anderson, Gerard. 1985a. "National Medical Care Spending." *Health Affairs*, 4, 3: 100–107.

Anderson, Gerard, and James Studnicki. 1985b. "Insurers Competing with Providers." *Hospitals* 59, 23: 64–66.

Anderson, Gerard. 1986. "National Medical Care Spending." *Health Affairs* 5, 3: 123–130.

Arbitman, Deborah. 1986. "A Primer on Patient Classification Systems and Their Relevance to Ambulatory Care." *Journal of Ambulatory Care Management* 9, 1: 58–81.

Cassidy, Robert. 1983. "Will the PPO Movement Freeze You Out?" *Medical Economics*, 18 April, pp. 262–274.

Davis, Karen, Gerard Anderson, Steven Renn, *et al.* 1985. "Is Cost Containment Working?" *Health Affairs* 4, 3: 81–94.

Eisenberg, John, and Deborah Kitz. 1986. "Savings from Outpatient Antibiotic Therapy for Osteomyelitis: Economic Analysis of a Therapeutic Strategy." *JAMA* 255, 12: 1584–1588.

Fitzgerald, John, Leonard Fagan, William Tierney, and Robert Dittus. 1987. "Changing Patterns of Hip Fracture Care Before and After Implementation of the Prospective Payment System." *JAMA* 258, 2: 218–221.

Folse, Lynn. 1985. "Alternative Sites Offer New Options for Consumers." *Advertising Age*, October 24.

Freedman, Steven. 1985. "Megacorporate Health Care: A Choice for the Future." *NEnglJMed* 312, 9: 579–582.

Fuchs, Victor. 1986. "Has Cost Containment Gone Too Far?" *Milbank Quarterly* 64, 3: 479–488.

Gabel, Jon, and Dan Ermann. 1985. "Preferred Provider Organizations: Performance, Problems, and Promise." *Health Affairs* 4, 1: 24–40.

Gabel, Jon, Dan Ermann, Thomas Rice, and Greg deLissovoy. 1986. "The

Emergence and Future of PPOs." *Journal of Health Politics, Policy and Law* 11, 2: 305–322.

Gabel, Jon, Cindy Jajich-Toth, Karen Williams, *et al.* 1987. "The Commercial Health Insurance Industry in Transition." *Health Affairs* 6, 3: 46–60.

Ginzberg, Eli. 1985. "The Restructuring of U.S. Health Care." *Inquiry* 22, 3: 272–281.

Ginzberg, Eli. 1986. "The Destabilization of Health Care." *NEnglJMed* 315, 12: 757–761.

Gray, Bradford, and Walter McNerney. 1986. "For-Profit Enterprise in Health Care: The Institute of Medicine Study." *NEnglJMed* 314, 23: 1523–1528.

Iglehart, John. 1985. "U.S. Health Care System: A Look to the 1990s." *Health Affairs* 4, 3: 120–127.

Iglehart, John. 1986. "Early Experience with Prospective Payment of Hospitals." *NEnglJMed* 314, 22: 1460–1464.

Koren, Mary Jane. 1986. "Home Care—Who Cares?" *NEnglJMed* 314, 14: 917–920.

Lawrence, Jean. 1984. "Demand the Right Not to Wait for a Doctor." *Washington Post*, July 22.

Lefton, Doug. 1985. "Hospitals Score Record Profits under DRGs." *American Medical News*, August 9.

Luft, Harold. 1981. *Health Maintenance Organizations: Dimensions of Performance.* New York: Wiley.

Milligan, John. 1985. "Showdown at Medicine Bend." *Institutional Investor*, October, pp. 225–227.

Moxley, John, and Penelope Roeder. 1984. "New Opportunities for Out-of-Hospital Health Services." *NEnglJMed* 310, 3: 193–197.

"New Sites for Care and Cure." 1985. *New York Times*, Supplement: "Health and Medicine Employment Outlook," November 3, p. 15.

Relman, Arnold. 1980. "The New Medical-Industrial Complex." *NEnglJMed* 303, 17: 963–970.

Richards, Glenn. 1984. "FECs Pose Competition for Hospital EDs: Freestanding Emergency Centers Doubling in Number Yearly." *Hospitals* 58, 6: 77–82.

Saward, Ernest, and E. K. Gallagher. 1983. "Reflections on Change in Medical Practice: The Current Trend to Large-Scale Medical Organizations." *JAMA* 250, 20: 2820–2825.

Scheier, Ronni. 1986. "HMO Enrollment Drops for First Time." *American Medical News*, January 10.

Smego, Raymond. 1985. "Home Intravenous Antibiotic Therapy." *Archives of Internal Medicine* 145, 6: 1001–1002.

Steinwachs, Donald, Jonathan Weiner, Paul Batalden, Kathy Coltin, and Fred Wasserman. 1986. "A Comparison of the Requirements for Primary Care Physicians in HMOs with Projections Made by the GMENAC." *NEnglJMed* 314, 4: 217–222.

U.S. General Accounting Office. 1985. *Constraining National Health Care Expenditures: Achieving Quality Care at an Affordable Cost.* Pub. GAO/HRD-85-105. Washington, D.C.: GPO.

Weiner, Jonathan. 1986. "Assuring Quality of Care in HMOs: Past Lessons, Present Challenges and Future Directions." *Journal of the Group Health Association of America* 7: 10–27.

Chapter 9

AMA. 1987. *The Health Policy Agenda for the American People; Final Report*. Chicago: AMA.

Beauchamp, Tom, and James Childress. 1983. *Principles of Biomedical Ethics*, 2nd ed. New York: Oxford University Press.

Bovbjerg, Randall, Philip Held, and Louis Diamond. 1987. "Provider-Patient Relations and Treatment Choice in the Era of Fiscal Incentives: The Case of the End-Stage Renal Disease Program." *Milbank Quarterly* 65, 2: 177–202.

Colombotos, John, and Corinne Kirchner. 1986. *Physicians and Social Change*. New York: Oxford University Press.

Eisenberg, John, and Sankey Williams. 1981. "Cost Containment and Changing Physicians' Practice Behavior: Can the Fox Learn to Guard the Chicken Coop?" *JAMA* 246, 19: 2195–2201.

Hammarskjöld, Dag. 1980. *Markings*. New York: Alfred A. Knopf.

Iglehart, John. 1984. "Opinion Polls on Health Care." *NEnglJMed* 310, 24: 1616–1620.

King, Lester. 1985. "Medicine—Trade or Profession." *JAMA* 253, 18: 2709–2710.

Kramon, Glenn. 1988. "Insurance Rates for Health Care Increase Sharply." *New York Times*, January 12, p. 1.

Louis Harris and Associates. 1983. *The Equitable Healthcare Survey: Options for Controlling Costs*.

Louis Harriss and Associates, 1984. *The Equitable Healthcare Survey II: Physicians' Attitudes Toward Cost Containment*.

Prather, Hugh. 1970. *Notes to Myself*. Moab, Utah: Real People Press.

Relman, Arnold. 1983. "The Future of Medical Practice." *Health Affairs* 2, 2: 5–19.

Relman, Arnold. 1985. "Cost Control, Doctors' Ethics, and Patient Care." *Issues in Science and Technology*, Winter, pp. 103–111.

Thomasma, David, Kenneth Micetich, and Patricia Steinecker. 1985. "Social Censorship of Medical and Ethical Decisions." *The Pharos* 48, 3: 22–26.

Thurow, Lester. 1984. "Learning to Say No." *NEnglJMed* 311, 24: 1569–1572.

Young, David. 1985. "Physician Accountability for Health Care Costs." *Business and Health*, November, pp. 16–18.

Chapter 10

AMA. 1986a. *Physician Characteristics and Distribution in the U.S.* Chicago: AMA.

AMA. 1986b. *Socioeconomic Characteristcs of Medical Practice 1986*. Chicago: AMA.

Angell, Marcia. 1985. "Cost Containment and the Physician." *JAMA* 254, 9: 1203–1207.

Berger, Stanley, and Amy Roth. 1984. "Prospective Payment and the University Hospital." *NEnglJMed* 310, 5: 316–318.

Breo, Dennis. 1985. "Band Together or Lose Professional Freedom, Physicians Warned." *American Medical News*, July 19, pp. 2, 19–21.

Brook, Robert, and Kathleen Lohr. 1985. "Efficiency, Effectiveness, Variations, and Quality: Boundary-Crossing Research." *Medical Care* 23, 5: 710–722.

Cameron, James. 1985. "The Indirect Costs of Graduate Medical Education." *NEnglJMed* 312, 19: 1233–1238.

Daniels, Norman. 1986. "Why Saying No to Patients in the United States Is So Hard: Cost Containment, Justice, and Provider Autonomy." *NEnglJMed* 314, 21: 1380–1383.

Des Harnais, Susan, Edward Kobrinski, James Chesney, *et al.* 1987. "The Early Effects of the Prospective Payment System on Inpatient Utilization and the Quality of Care." *Inquiry* 24, 1: 7–16.

Dolenc, Danielle, and Charles Dougherty. 1985. "DRGs: The Counterrevolution in Financing Health Care." *Hastings Center Report* 15, 3: 19–29.

Durenburger, David. 1985. "Who, How, and When to Pay for Physicians' Training." *Business and Health*, April, pp. 7–11.

Dyer, Allen. 1986. "Patients, Not Costs, Come First." *Hastings Center Report* 16, 1: 5–7.

Elstein, Arthur. 1985. "Consultation and Referral in New Medical-Practice Environments: A Gloomy Outlook?" *Annals of Internal Medicine* 85, 4: 616–617.

Fineberg, Harvey, 1985. "Future Directions for Research." *Medical Decision Making* 5, 1: 35–38.

Ginzberg, Eli. 1983. "Cost Containment—Imaginary and Real." *NEnglJMed* 308, 20: 1220–1224.

Gray, Bradford, ed. 1986. *For-Profit Enterprise in Health Care.* A publication of the National Academy of Science, Institute of Medicine. Washington, D.C.: National Academy Press.

Herzlinger, Regina, and William Krasker. 1987. "Who Profits from Non-Profits?" *Harvard Business Review*, January-February, pp. 93–106.

Horn, Susan, Phoebe Sharkey, Angela Chambers, and Roger Horn. 1985. "Severity of Illness Within DRGs: Impact on Prospective Payment." *AmJPubHealth* 75, 10: 1195–1199.

Iglehart, John. 1986. "Early Experience with Prospective Payment of Hospitals." *NEnglJMed* 314, 22: 1460–1464.

Juba, David. 1985. "Medicare Part B: A Time for Reform." *Business and Health*, November, pp. 5–8.

Kahn, Henry, and Peter Orris. 1982. "The Emerging Role of Salaried Physicians: An Organizational Proposal." *Journal of Public Health Policy* 3, 3: 284–292.

King, Lester. 1985. "Medicine—Trade or Profession?" *JAMA* 253, 18: 2709–2710.

Korcok, Milan. 1986. "From Patient Advocate to 'Gatekeeper.'" *American Medical News*, April 4, pp. 21–23.

Levinsky, Norman. 1984. "The Doctor's Master." *NEnglJMed* 311, 24: 1573–1575.

Loewy, Erich. 1980. "Should Cost Be a Factor in Personal Medical Care?" Letter to the Editor. *NEnglJMed* 303, 5: 288.

Lowenstein, Steven, Lisa Iezzoni, and Mark Moskowitz. 1985. "Prospective Payment for Physician Services: Impact on Medical Consultation Practices." *JAMA* 254, 18: 2632–2637.

Ludmerer, Kenneth. 1985. *Learning to Heal: The Development of American Medical Education.* New York: Basic Books.

Luft, Harold. 1982. "Health Maintenance Organizations and the Rationing of Medical Care." *Milbank Memorial Fund Quarterly* 60, 2: 268–306.

Morreim, E. Haavi. 1985. "The MD and the DRG." *Hastings Center Report* 15, 3: 30–38.

National Academy of Sciences, Institute of Medicine. 1985. *Assessing Medical Technologies*. Washington, D.C.: National Academy Press.

Nutter, Donald. 1984. "Access to Care and the Evolution of Corporate, For-Profit Medicine." *NEnglJMed* 311, 14: 917–919.

Omenn, Gilbert, and Douglas Conrad. 1984. "Implications of DRGs for Clinicians." *NEnglJMed* 311, 20: 1314–1317.

Petersdorf, Robert. 1985. "Current and Future Directions for Hospital and Physician Reimbursement: Effect on the Academic Medical Center." *JAMA* 253, 17: 2543–2548.

Rabkin, Mitchell. 1982. "The SAG Index." *NEnglJMed* 307, 21: 1350–1351.

Reinhardt, Uwe. 1982. "Table Manners at the Health Care Feast." In *Financing Health Care: Competition Vs. Regulation*, edited by Duncan Yaggy and William Anylan, pp. 13–34. Cambridge, Mass.: Ballinger Publishing.

Relman, Arnold. 1980. "The New Medical-Industrial Complex." *NEnglJMed* 303, 17: 963–970.

Rock, Robert. 1985. "Assuring Quality of Care under DRG-Based Prospective Payment." *Medical Decision Making* 5, 1: 31–34.

Saward, Ernest, and E. K. Gallagher. "Reflections on Change in Medical Practice: The Current Trend to Large-Scale Medical Organizations." *JAMA* 350, 20: 2820–2825.

Schroeder, James, John Clarke, and James Webster. 1985. "Prepaid Entitlements: A New Challenge for Physician-Patient Relationships." *JAMA* 254, 21: 3080–3082.

Shortell, Stephen, Michael Morrisey, and Douglas Conrad. 1985. "Economic Regulation and Hospital Behavior: The Effects on Medical Staff Organization and Hospital-Physician Relationships." *Health Services Research* 20, 5: 597–628.

Simborg, Donald. 1981. "DRG Creep: A New Hospital-Acquired Disease." *NEnglJMed* 304, 26: 1602–1604.

Smits, Helen, and Rita Watson. 1984. "DRGs and the Future of Surgical Practice." *NEnglJMed* 311, 25: 1612–1615.

Steinwald, Bruce. 1986. "The Impact of New Reimbursement Schemes on Clinical Research in Hospitals: The Case of the Prospective Payment System." *Journal of General Internal Medicine* 1, supplement: S56–S59.

Swick, Thomas. 1986. "The Emergence of Physician Unions . . . Can They Balance Economic and Public Interests?" *American College of Physicians Observer*, March, pp. 4–5.

Thomasma, David, Kenneth Micetich, and Patricia Steinecker. 1985. "Social Censorship of Medical and Ethical Decisions." *The Pharos* 48, 3: 22–26.

Thurow, Lester. 1984. "Learning to Say No." *NEnglJMed* 311, 24: 1569–1572.

Veatch, Robert. 1986. "DRGs and the Ethical Allocation of Resources." *Hastings Center Report* 16, 3: 32–40.

Wennberg, John, Klim McPherson, and Philip Capter. 1984. "Will Payment Based on Diagnosis-Related Groups Control Hospital Costs?" *NEnglJMed* 311, 5: 295–300.

Williams, Sankey. 1985. "The Impact of DRG-Based Prospective Payment on Clinical Decision Making." *Medical Decision Making* 5, 2: 23–29.

Yarbro, J. W., and L. E. Mortenson. 1985. "The Need for Diagnosis-Related Group 471: Protection for Clinical Research." *JAMA* 253, 5: 684–685.
Young, David, and Richard Saltman. 1985. *The Hospital Power Equilibrium: Physician Behavior and Cost Control*. Baltimore: Johns Hopkins University Press.

Chapter 11

Charache, Samuel, Lydia Nelson, Edward Keyser, and Paul Metzger. 1985. "A Clinical Trial of Three-Part Electronic Differential White Blood Cell Counts." *Archives of Internal Medicine* 145; 10: 1852–1855.
Close, Pamela. 1984. "Economic Changes Affecting Medical Practice: What Do Medical Students Need to Know?" *OSR Report* 8, no. 1.
Daniels, Marcia, and Steven Schroeder. 1977. "Variations among Physicians in Use of Laboratory Tests II. Relation to Clinical Productivity and Outcomes of Care." *Medical Care* 15, 6: 482–487.
Dans, Peter, Jonathan Weiner, Jacques Milan, and Lewis Becker. 1983. "Conditional Probability in the Diagnosis of Coronary Artery Disease: Implications for Eliminating Unnecessary Testing." *Southern Medical Journal* 76, pp. 1118–1121.
Dans, Peter. 1985. "Cost-Effective Management of Pneumonia." *Hospital Therapy*, November, pp. 23–44.
Donabedian, Avedis. 1980. *Explorations in Quality Assessment and Monitoring*, vol. 1: *The Definition of Quality and Approaches to Its Assessment*. Ann Arbor, Mich.: Health Administration Press.
Eddy, David. 1984. "Variations in Physician Practice: The Role of Uncertainty." *Health Affairs* 3, 2: 74–89.
Egdahl, Richard, and Cynthia Taft. 1986. "Financial Incentives to Physicians." *NEnglJMed* 315, 1: 59–61.
Eisenberg, John. 1986a. *Doctors' Decisions and the Cost of Medical Care*. Ann Arbor, Mich.: Health Administration Press.
Eisenberg, John, and Deborah Kitz. 1986b. "Savings from Outpatient Antibiotic Therapy for Osteomyelitis: Economic Analysis of a Therapeutic Strategy." *JAMA* 255, 12: 1584–1588.
Estaugh, Steven. 1981. "Teaching the Principles of Cost-Effective Clinical Decisionmaking to Medical Students." *Inquiry* 18, 1: 28–36.
Fineberg, Harvey. 1985. "Technology Assessment: Motivation, Capability, and Future Directions." *Medical Care* 23, 5: 663–671.
Fryback, Dennis. 1985. "Decision Maker, Quantify Thyself!" *Medical Decision Making* 5, 1: 51–60.
Fuchs, Victor. 1974. *Who Shall Live? Health, Economics, and Social Choice*. New York: Basic Books.
Ginzberg, Eli. 1986. "The Destabilization of Health Care." *NEnglJMed* 315, 12: 757–761.
HCFA. 1986. *The Medicare and Medicaid Data Book, 1984*. HCFA Pub. No. 03210. Baltimore.
Hubbell, F. Allan, Sheldon Greenfield, Judy Tyler, *et al.* 1985. "The Impact of Routine Admission Chest X-Ray Films on Patient Care." *NEnglJMed* 312, 4: 209–213.

Huth, Edward. 1985. "Needed: An Economics Approach to Systems for Medical Information." *Annals of Internal Medicine* 103, 4: 617–619.

Iglehart, John. 1986. "Early Experience with Prospective Payment of Hospitals." *NEnglJMed* 314, 22: 1460–1464.

Klinefelter, Harry. 1982. "The Mixed-Blessing of Technology." *The Internist*, March, pp. 9–10.

Komaroff, Anthony. 1985. "Quality Assurance in 1984." *Medical Care* 23, 5: 723–734.

Ludmerer, Kenneth. 1985. *Learning to Heal: The Development of American Medical Education*. New York: Basic Books.

MacKenzie, C. Ronald, Mary Charlson, Denise DiGioia, and Kathleen Kelley. 1986. "A Patient-Specific Measure of Change in Maximal Function." *Archives of Internal Medicine* 146, 7: 1325–1329.

McCarthy, Eugene, Madelon Finkel, and Hirsch Ruchlin. 1981. "Second Opinions on Elective Surgery." *Lancet*, June 20, 1352–1354.

McNeil, Barbara. 1985. "Hospital Response to DRG-Based Prospective Payment." *Medical Decision Making* 5, 1: 15–21.

McPherson, Klim, John Wennberg, Ole Hovind, and Peter Clifford. 1982. "Small-Area Variations in the Use of Common Surgical Procedures: An International Comparison of New England, England, and Norway." *NEnglJMed* 307, 21: 1310–1314.

Morreim, E. Haavi. 1985. "The MD and the DRG." *Hastings Center Report* 15, 3: 30–38.

National Academy of Sciences, Institute of Medicine. 1985. *Assessing Medical Technologies*. Washington, D.C.: National Academy Press.

Perry, Seymour. 1986. "Technology Assessment: Continuing Uncertainty." *NEnglJMed* 314, 4: 240–243.

President's Commission for the Study of Ethical Problems in Medicine and Biomedical and Behavioral Research. 1982. USGPO-1982-0383-515/8673.

Pryor, David, Robert Califf, Frank Harrell, *et al.* 1985. "Clinical Data Bases: Accomplishments and Unrealized Potential." *Medical Care* 23, 5: 623–647.

Reinhardt, Uwe. 1985. "Future Trends in the Economics of Medical Practice and Care." *AmJCardiology* 56, 5: 50C–59C.

Relman, Arnold. 1980. "Assessment of Medical Practices: A Simple Proposal." *NEnglJMed* 303, 3: 153–154.

Relman, Arnold. 1985. "Cost Control, Doctors' Ethics and Patient Care." *Issues in Science and Technology*, Winter, pp. 103–111.

Rhyne, Robert, and Stephen Gehlbach. 1979. "Effects of an Educational Feedback Strategy on Physician Utilization of Thyroid Function Panels." *Journal of Family Practice* 8, 5: 1003–1007.

Robin, Eugene. 1985. "The Cult of the Swan-Ganz Catheter: Overuse and Abuse of Pulmonary Flow Catheters." *Annals of Internal Medicine* 103, 3: 445–449.

Shortliffe, Edward. 1987. "Computer Programs to Support Clinical Decision Making." *JAMA* 258, 1: 61–66.

Showstack, Jonathan, Mary Stone, and Steven Schroeder. 1985. "The Role of Changing Clinical Practices in the Rising Costs of Hospital Care." *NEnglJMed* 313, 19: 1201–1207.

Stern, Robert, and Arnold Epstein. 1985. "Institutional Responses to Prospective Payment Based on Diagnosis-Related Groups: Implications for Cost, Quality, and Access." *NEnglJMed* 312, 10: 621–627.

Tobin, Richard. 1980. "Should Cost Be a Factor in Personal Medical Care?" Letter to the Editor. *NEnglJMed* 303, 5: 288.

USDHHS, National Center for Devices and Radiological Health. 1983. *The Selection of Patients for X-Ray Examinations: Chest X-Ray Screening Examinations.* HHS (FDA) 83-8204. Washington, D.C.: GPO.

Walsh, Diana, and Richard Egdahl. 1977. *Payer, Provider, Consumer: Industry Confronts Health Care Costs.* New York: Springer-Verlag.

Wasson, John, Harold Sox, Raymond Neff, and Lee Goldman. 1985. "Clinical Prediction Rules: Applications and Methodological Standards." *NEnglJMed* 313, 13: 793–799.

Weinstein, Milton, and William Stason. 1977. "Foundations of Cost-Effectiveness Analysis for Health and Medical Practices." *NEnglJMed* 296, 13: 716–721.

Wennberg, John, and Alan Gittelsohn. 1982. "Variations in Medical Care Among Small Areas." *Scientific American* 246: 4: 120–132.

Wennberg, John. 1985. "On Patient Need, Equity, Supplier-Induced Demand, and the Need to Assess the Outcome of Common Medical Practices." *Medical Care* 23, 5: 512–520.

Young, David. 1985. "Physician Accountability for Health Care Costs." *Business and Health*, November, pp. 16–18.

Chapter 12

AMA. 1986. *Socioeconomic Characteristics of Medical Practice 1986.* Chicago: AMA.

AMA, Special Task Force on Professional Liability and Insurance. 1984. *Professional Liability in the '80s*, Reports 1–3. Chicago: AMA.

"AMA Statement Rebuts Claims by Trial Lawyers' Association." 1985. *American Medical News*, October 4, pp. 36–39.

Anderson, Eugene. 1986. "Compensation, Without Lawyers." *New York Times*, May 1, p. Y29.

Angell, Marcia. 1985. "Cost Containment and the Physician." *JAMA* 254, 9: 1203–1207.

Baily, Mary Ann, and Warren Cikins, eds. 1985. *The Effects of Litigation on Health Care Costs.* Washington, D.C.: Brookings Institution.

Bosk, Charles. 1986. "Professional Responsibility and Medical Error." In *Applications of Social Science to Clinical Medicine and Health Policy*, edited by Linda Aiken and David Mechanic, pp. 460–477. New Brunswick, N.J.: Rutgers University Press.

Bovbjerg, Randall, and Clark Havighurst. 1985. "Medical Malpractice: An Update for Noncombatants." *Business and Health*, September, pp. 38–42.

Crane, Mark. 1986. "Malpractice: The Most Dangerous Places to Practice." *Medical Economics*, February 3, pp. 65–71.

"Doctors and Lawyers Square Off on Lawsuits." 1985. *New York Times*, December 26.

Dolin, Leigh. 1985. "Antitrust Law Versus Peer Review." *NEnglJMed* 313, 18: 1156–1157.

Henderson, Charles. 1986. "A Medical Malpractice Primer." *Maryland Medical Journal* 35, 1: 38–42.

Hunter, Robert. 1986. "Taming the Latest Insurance 'Crisis.'" *New York Times*, April 13, p. F3.

"Insurance Monitor." 1986. *Maryland Medical Journal* 35, 1: 10.

Jury Verdict Research. 1985. *Current Award Trends*, January. Solon, Ohio.

Lee, Richard. 1986. "The Jaundiced View: Malpractice Malaise." *American Journal of Medicine* 80, 2: 159–160.

O'Connell, Jeffrey. 1985. "The Case Against the Current Malpractice System." Presentation at The Urban Institute's National Medical Malpractice Conference, "Can the Private Sector Find Relief?" February 21–22, 1985.

Pauker, Stephen, and Jerome Kassirer. 1987. "Decision Analysis." *NEnglJMed* 316, 5: 250–258.

Rust, Mark. 1985. "MDs Cease High-Risk Care in N.Y." *American Medical News*, June 21, pp. 1, 26.

Rust, Mark. 1986a. "MDs No Longer Alone in Tort Reform Fight." *American Medical News*, February 14, pp. 1, 23, 25, 26.

Rust, Mark. 1986b. "Tort Reform Legislation Gains Momentum." *American Medical News*, April 25, pp. 1, 28, 29.

Rust, Mark. 1987. "Malpractice: New Alliances Aid in Passage of Tort Reforms." *American Medical News*, January 2, pp. 3, 35.

Schwartz, William, and Henry Aaron. 1984. "Rationing Hospital Care: Lessons from Britain." *NEnglJMed* 310, 1: 52–56.

Siden, Harold, Benjamin Ticho, and Mitchell Kopnick. 1986. "Malpractice Concerns Enter the Medical School Classroom." Letter to the Editor. *NEnglJMed* 314, 8: 522–523.

Stempfer, Meir, Walter Willet, Graham Colditz, *et al.* 1985. "A Prospective Study of Postmenopausal Estrogen Therapy and Coronary Heart Disease." *NEnglJMed* 313, 17: 1044–1049.

Williams, Sarah, ed. 1985. "Medical Malpractice Resurfacing as Issue for States." *Alpha Centerpiece*, October. Washington, D.C. (HCFA Grant #18-P-9814/3-03).

Wilson, Peter, Robert Garrison, and William Castelli. 1985. "Postmenopausal Estrogen Use, Cigarette Smoking, and Cardiovascular Morbidity in Women over 50: The Framingham Study." *NEnglJMed* 313, 17: 1038–1043.

Chapter 13

Aday, Lu Ann, and Ronald Anderson. 1975. *Access to Medical Care*. Ann Arbor, Mich.: Health Administration Press.

Annas, George. 1986. "Your Money or Your Life: 'Dumping' Uninsured Patients from Hospital Emergency Wards." *AmJPubHealth* 76, 1: 74–77.

Berman, Neal, and Phyllis Lauro. 1985. "Determining the True Cost of Graduate Medical Education." *Business and Health*, April, pp. 12–13.

Blendon, Robert, Linda Aiken, Howard Freeman, *et al.* 1986. "Uncompensated Care by Hospitals or Public Insurance for the Poor: Does It Make a Difference?" *NEnglJMed* 314, 18: 1160–1163.

Blumenthal, David, Mark Schlesinger, Pamela Drumheller, and The Harvard Medicare Project. 1986. "The Future of Medicare." *NEnglJMed* 314, 11: 722–728.

Brandon, William. 1982. "Health-Related Tax Subsidies: Government Handouts for the Affluent." *NEnglJMed* 307, 15: 947–950.

Brook, Robert, John Ware, William Rogers, *et al.* 1983. "Does Free Care Improve Adults' Health?: Results from a Randomized Controlled Trial." *NEnglJMed* 309, 23: 1426–1434.

Calkins, David, Linda Burns, and Thomas Delbanco. 1986. "Ambulatory Care and the Poor: Tracking the Impact of Changes in Federal Policy." *Journal of General Internal Medicine* 1, 2: 109–115.

Citrin, Toby. 1985. "Trustees at the Focal Point." *NEnglJMed* 313, 19: 1223–1226.

Daniels, Norman. 1986. "Why Saying No to Patients in the United States Is So Hard: Cost Containment, Justice, and Provider Autonomy." *NEnglJMed* 314, 21: 1380–1383.

Davidson, Stephen, Jerry Cromwell, and Rachel Shurman. 1986. "Medicaid Myths: Trends in Medicaid Expenditures and the Prospects for Reform." *Journal of Health Politics, Policy and Law* 10, 4: 699–728.

Davis, Karen, and Cathy Schoen. 1978. *Health and the War on Poverty: A Ten-Year Appraisal.* Washington, D.C.: Brookings Institution.

Davis, Karen. 1985. "Access to Health Care: A Matter of Fairness." In *Health Care: How to Improve It and Pay for It,* pp. 45–57. Washington, D.C.: Center for National Policy.

Ginsburg, Paul, and Frank Sloan. 1984. "Hospital Cost Shifting." *NEnglJMed* 310, 14: 893–898.

Health Policy Alternatives. 1985. "Paying for Physicians' Services under Medicare: Issues and Reform Options for the American Association of Retired Persons." A report to the American Association of Retired Persons on Medicare Physician Payment Reform.

Iglehart, John. 1985. "U.S. Health Care System: A Look to the 1990s." *Health Affairs* 4, 3: 120–127.

Johns, Lucy. 1985. "Selective Contracting in California." *Health Affairs* 4, 3: 32–48.

Jolly, Paul, Leon Taskel, and David Baime. 1986. "U.S. Medical School Finances." *JAMA* 256, 12: 1570–1580.

King, Wayne. 1985. "Texas Adopts Stringent Rules on Rights of Poor at Hospitals." *New York Times,* December 15, p. 30.

Louis Harris and Associates. 1984. *The Equitable Healthcare Survey II: Physicians' Attitudes Toward Cost Containment.*

Lurie, Nicole, Nancy Ward, Martin Shapiro, and Robert Brook. 1984. "Termination from Medi-Cal—Does It Affect Health?" *NEnglJMed* 311, 7: 480–484.

National Center for Health Services Research. 1980. "Who Are the Uninsured?" Data Preview 1 from the National Health Care Expenditures Study, Public Health Service, Department of Health and Human Services. Washington, D.C.

Navarro, Vicente. 1987. "Federal Health Policies in the United States: An Alternative Explanation." *Milbank Quarterly* 65, 1: 81–111.

Nutter, Donald. 1984. "Access to Care and the Evolution of Corporate, For-Profit Medicine." *NEnglJMed* 311, 14: 917–919.

Penchansky, Roy, and J. William Thomas. 1981. "The Concept of Access: Definition and Relationship to Consumer Satisfaction." *Medical Care* 19, 2: 127–140.

Reinhardt, Uwe. 1986. "Rationing the Nation's Health-Care Surplus: A Paradox? or As American as Apple Pie?" Statement before The House Select Committee on Aging, United States Congress. Washington, D.C.

Relman, Arnold, and Uwe Reinhardt. 1986. "Debating For-Profit Health Care." *Health Affairs* 5, 2: 5–31.

Richards, Glenn. 1984. "FECs Pose Competition for Hospital EDs." *Hospitals* 58, 6: 77–82.

Robert Wood Johnson Foundation. 1987. *Access to Health Care in the U.S.* Special Report No. 2.

Scheier, Ronni. 1986a. "Hospital's Burden: The Rising Uninsured." *American Medical News*, April 4, pp. 3, 39–40.

Scheier, Ronni. 1986b. "States Continue Expansion of Medicaid Programs." *American Medical News*, May 9, p. 9.

Schiff, Robert, David Ansell, James Schlosser, *et al.* 1986. "Transfers to a Public Hospital: A Prospective Study of 467 Patients." *NEnglJMed* 314, 9: 552–557.

Schramm, Carl. 1983. "The Teaching Hospital and the Future Role of State Government." *NEnglJMed* 308, 1: 41–45.

Sloan, Frank, James Blumstein, and James Perrin, eds. 1986. *Uncompensated Hospital Care: Rights and Responsibilities*. Baltimore: Johns Hopkins University Press.

Sulvetta, Margaret, and Katherine Swartz. 1986. *The Uninsured and Uncompensated Care*. National Health Policy Forum. Washington, D.C.

USDHHS. 1986. *Health of the Disadvantaged*. DHHS Pub #HRS-P-DV86-2.

Washington News Letter. 1985. Published by the American Public Health Association. No. 9. Washington, D.C.

Chapter 14

Aaron, Henry, and William Schwartz. 1984. *The Painful Prescription*. Washington, D.C.: Brookings Institution.

Angell, Marcia. 1985. "Cost Containment and the Physician." *JAMA* 254, 9: 1203–1207.

Annas, George. 1986. "Your Money or Your Life: 'Dumping' Uninsured Patients from Hospital Emergency Wards." *AmJPubHealth* 76, 1: 74–77.

Bayer, Ronald, Daniel Callahan, John Fletcher, *et al.* 1983. "The Care of the Terminally Ill: Morality and Economics." *NEnglJMed* 309, 24: 1490–1494.

Bennett, Ivan. 1977. "Technology as Shaping Force." In *Doing Better and Feeling Worse: Health in the United States*, edited by John Knowles, pp. 125–133. New York: W. W. Norton.

Blainpain, Jan. 1985. "The Changing Environment of Health Care." *International Journal of Technology Assessment in Health Care* 1, 2: 271–277.

Blendon, Robert, and David Rogers. 1983. "Cutting Medical Care Costs: *Primum Non Nocere*." *JAMA* 250, 14: 1880–1885.

Blendon, Robert, and Drew Altman. 1984. "Public Attitudes about Health-Care Costs: A Lesson in National Schizophrenia." *NEnglJMed* 311, 9: 613–616.

Brook, Robert, and Kathleen Lohr. 1986. "Will We Need to Ration Effective Health Care?" *Issues in Science and Technology*, Fall, pp. 68–77.

Callahan, Daniel. 1987. *Setting Limits: Medical Goals in an Aging Society*. New York: Simon and Schuster.

Calmes, Selma. 1984. "Memories of Polio." *Archives of Internal Medicine* 144, 6: 1273.

Daniels, Norman. 1985. *Just Health Care.* New York: Cambridge University Press.

Daniels, Norman. 1986. "Why Saying No to Patients in the United States Is So Hard: Cost Containment, Justice, and Provider Autonomy." *NEnglJMed* 314, 21: 1380–1383.

Davis, William. 1986. "'THEY' Threaten Medical System." *American Medical News,* September 5, p. 29.

Dolenc, Danielle, and Charles Dougherty. 1985. "DRGs: The Counterrevolution in Financing Health Care." *Hastings Center Report* 15, 3: 19–29.

Donabedian, Avedis. 1980. *Explorations in Quality Assessment and Monitoring,* vol. 1: *The Definition of Quality and Approaches to Its Assessment.* Ann Arbor, Mich.: Health Administration Press.

Eisenberg, Carola. 1986. "It Is Still a Privilege to Be a Doctor." *NEnglJMed* 314, 17: 1113–1114.

Foege, William, Robert Amler, and Craig White. 1985. "Closing the Gap: Report of the Carter Center Health Policy Consultation." *JAMA* 254, 10: 1355–1358.

Fuchs, Victor. 1984. "The Rationing of Medical Care." *NEnglJMed* 311, 24: 1572–1573.

Fuchs, Victor. 1986. "Has Cost Containment Gone Too Far?" *Milbank Quarterly* 64, 3: 479–488.

Iglehart, John. 1984. "Opinion Polls on Health Care." *NEnglJMed* 310, 24: 1616–1620.

Iglehart, John. 1986. "Early Experience with Prospective Payment of Hospitals." *NEnglJMed* 314, 22: 1460–1464.

King, Lester. 1985. "Medicine—Trade or Profession?" *JAMA* 253, 18: 2709–2710.

Levinsky, Norman. 1984. "The Doctor's Master." *NEnglJMed* 311, 24: 1573–1575.

Lewis, Irving, and Cecil Sheps. 1983. *The Sick Citadel.* Cambridge, Mass.: Oelgeschlager, Gunn and Hain.

Lind, Stuart. 1986. "Fee-For-Service Research." *NEnglJMed* 314, 5: 312–315.

Loewy, Erich. 1980. "Cost Should Not Be a Factor in Medical Care." Letter to the Editor. *NEnglJMed* 302, 12: 697.

Louis Harris and Associates. 1983. *The Equitable Healthcare Survey: Options for Controlling Costs.*

Louis Harris and Associates. 1984. *The Equitable Healthcare Survey II: Physicians' Attitudes Toward Cost Containment.*

Ludmerer, Kenneth. 1985. *Learning to Heal: The Development of American Medical Education.* New York: Basic Books.

Miller, Frances, and Graham Miller. 1986. "The Painful Prescription: A Procrustean Perspective?" *NEnglJMed* 314, 21: 1383–1386.

O'Day, Steven. 1984. "The Hospice Movement: An Alternative to Euthanasia." Unpublished.

Reed, David. 1980. "Should Cost Be a Factor in Personal Medical Care?" Letter to the Editor. *NEnglJMed* 303, 5: 288.

Reinhardt, Uwe. 1987. "Resource Allocation in Health Care: The Allocation of Lifestyles to Providers." *Milbank Quarterly* 65, 2: 153–176.

Schwartz, William, and Henry Aaron. 1984. "Rationing Hospital Care: Lessons from Britain." *NEnglJMed* 310, 1: 52–56.

Shenkin, Henry. 1986. *Clinical Practice and Cost Containment: A Physician's Perspective.* New York: Praeger Publishers.

Somers, Anne. 1986. "The Changing Demand for Health Services: A Historical Perspective and Some Thoughts for the Future." *Inquiry* 23, 4: 395–402.

Steinberg, Earl, Jane Sisk, and Katherine Locke. 1985. "X-Ray CT and Magnetic Resonance Imagers: Diffusion Patterns and Policy Issues." *NEnglJMed* 313, 14: 859–864.

Thurow, Lester, 1984. "Learning to Say No." *NEnglJMed* 311, 24: 1569–1572.

Veatch, Robert. 1986. "DRGs and the Ethical Allocation of Resources." *Hastings Center Report* 16, 3: 32–40.

Watts, Malcolm. 1985. "Dealing with a Stereotype." *American Medical News*, September 27, p. 4.

Weiner, Jonathan. 1987. "Primary Care Delivery in the U.S. and Four Northwest European Countries: Comparing the 'Corporatized' with the 'Socialized.'" *Milbank Quarterly* 65, 3: 426–461.

Wilensky, Gail. 1985. "Making Decisions on Rationing." *Business and Health*, November, pp. 36–38.

ACKNOWLEDGMENTS

We are grateful to the numerous people who assisted us in the preparation of this book. Many people at the Johns Hopkins Hospital, the Johns Hopkins Schools of Medicine and Public Health, and other institutions helped us identify and prioritize reams of material that formed the basis of this synthesis. These persons included Gerard Anderson, Ph.D., Richard Black, M.D., Bill Bleisch, John Boitnott, M.D., Mark Geraci, M.D., Paul McCauley, M.D., Robert Miller, M.D., Steven O'Day, M.D., Uwe Reinhardt, Ph.D., Robert Rock, M.D., James Studnicki, Sc.D., and Andrew Sumner, M.D.

The computer-generated graphics in this text were created by Ethan Weiner of the Graphix Shop, Alexandria, Virginia.

The grant from the National Fund for Medical Education that in part supported the development of this book was sponsored by the AT&T and BankAmerica Corporations.

For critiquing earlier drafts we thank Elizabeth Fee, Ph.D., Richard Frank, Ph.D., Harry Klinefelter, M.D., Laura Morlock, Ph.D., Marie Stoline, R.N., Mary Torchia, M.D., Richard Torchia, M.D., Daniel Hardesty, M.D., and two anonymous reviewers.

For supporting this project in diverse ways, we extend our thanks to Anders Richter and Jess Bell, our editors, Langford Kidd, M.D., Henry Seidel, M.D., the William Yates family, the Johns Hopkins Health Services Research and Development Center, and particularly our families.

A.S.
J.P.W.

INDEX